EPILEPSY: A PERSONAL APPROACH

"That it is a 'labor of love' is apparent with almost every word....It is exceedingly well done and should receive the commendation it deserves."
—**William S. Fields, M.D., Professor of Neurology, and Chairman, Department of Neuro-Oncology, University of Texas M.D. Anderson Hospital and Tumor Institute**

"Designed to give needed help to those who face the problem of lack of information, uncertainty where to get help, and fear. . . a useful tool."
—**Senator Sally Anne Staples, State of Minnesota Senate**

✳   ✳   ✳   ✳

NANCY CARLISLE SCHUMACHER has had epilepsy all her life, experiencing uncontrolled seizures. Despite her neurological dysfunction, she has participated fully (and joyfully) in the activities non-epileptics enjoy. In writing *Epilepsy: A Personal Approach*, Ms. Schumacher has reviewed medical background and treatment, conducted interviews with parents who openly share their experiences of living with epileptic children, and consulted with top medical and educational experts on this disorder.

EPILEPSY:

A
PERSONAL
APPROACH

NANCY CARLISLE SCHUMACHER

WARNER BOOKS

A Warner Communications Company

Dedicated to the memory of Jody, my stepmother

WARNER BOOKS EDITION

Copyright © 1985 by Schenkman Publishing Company, Inc.
All rights reserved. This book, or parts thereof, may not be
reproduced in any form without written permission from the
author.

This Warner Books Edition is published by arrangement with
Schenkman Publishing Company, Inc., 190 Concord Avenue,
Cambridge, MA 02138

Cover art by Anthony Russo

Warner Books, Inc.
666 Fifth Avenue
New York, N.Y. 10103

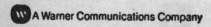 A Warner Communications Company

Printed in the United States of America

First Warner Books Printing: December, 1986

10 9 8 7 6 5 4 3 2 1

Here's To The Kids Who Are Different

Here's to the kids who are different;
The kids who don't always get A's
The kids who have ears,
Not at all like their peers
Or have noses that run on for days.

Here's to the kids who are different;
The kids who are just out of step.
The kids they all tease,
Who have cuts on their knees,
And whose sneakers are constantly wet.

Here's to the kids who are different;
The kids with a mischievous streak.
For when they are grown,
As history has shown,
It's their difference that makes them unique.

Digby Wolfe

ACLD NEWSBRIEFS—JULY/AUGUST 1978
BETTY LOU KRATOVILLE, EDITOR

Contents

Acknowledgements

F. J. L. Blasingame, M.D., Chicago, Illinois.

Daniel Halpern, University of Wisconsin Rehabilitation Center, Madison, Wisconsin.

Thomas E. Strax, M.D., Moss Rehabilitation Center, Philadelphia, PA.

Wm. S. Fields, M.D., University of Texas Medical School, Houston.

Fernando Torres, M.D., University of Minnesota Medical School, Minneapolis.

Joel Lubar, Ph.D., Department of Psychology, University of Tennessee.

W. W. Finley, M.D., Tulsa, Oklahoma.

M. B. Sterman, M.D., V. A. Hospital, Sepulvada, California.

Comprehensive Epilepsy Program, Minneapolis.

Epilepsy Foundation of America, Washington, D.C.

V. Elving Anderson, Deight Institute, University of Minnesota, Minneapolis.

Professeur Henri Gastaut, M.D., Groupe Hospitalier De La Timone, Marseille, Cedex 4, France.

Carol Banister, past director of the Minneapolis Epilepsy League.

Comprehensive Epilepsy Program personnel who lent their services.

Ann Schaerrer, editor of the *National Spokesman*, the newsletter for the Epilepsy Foundation of America.

Support of friends, family, especially my husband who had to put up with a great deal during the writing of this book; teachers and parents who were interviewed for this book.

Most especially, Bonnie Holtz who did the final editing of the manuscript.

Foreword

From the office of Senator Emily Anne Staples
STATE OF MINNESOTA, SENATE

Although in recent years resources for parents of children with special needs have multiplied, there is still a great deal of information left to be shared. This book, addressed specifically to the needs of children who have epilepsy, has been written for parents to identify community assistance of which they may otherwise be unaware.

Nancy Schumacher has been very thoughtful and painstaking in her efforts to locate and identify community resources which can play a significant role in helping these children lead normal, productive lives.

Recently, great strides have been made in the areas of education and employment. Through legislation passed at both the federal and state levels, greater access to education is mandated and programs designed to assist these children are required to be made available in every school district in the nation. Teachers are being given special training and parents are becoming more militant and organizing more effectively to secure the assistance that has been legislatively made available to them. As parents organize, they share information and help alleviate fears, as well as correct some of the myths people have about multiple sclerosis, epilepsy, or cerebral palsy.

While tools have been provided by legislation, there is unevenness in school districts working with these tools. The demand that they be used as they were designed must often come from parents or community advocates, particularly if the number to be served is few. Constant attention must be paid to see that those programs which should be made available *are* made available. In a time of tight budget prioritizing that is not always easy.

Employment is another area in which changes are being made. The non-discriminatory provisions of affirmative action legislation are more and more being interpreted to include those with cerebral palsy and epilepsy. Employers are learning how effectively these people can operate in a work situation and are becoming more willing to employ them. In this effort, too, education plays a critical role.

This book is designed to give needed help to those who face the problems of lack of information, uncertainty about where to get help, and fear. It should be a useful tool.

Sally Anne Staples

Preface

As a person who has had epilepsy all of my life, I feel that my personal experience enables me to approach the question of how to deal with epilepsy from a perspective different than that of the physician or the scientist. I have had epilepsy since I was two-and-one-half years old and have experienced every type of seizure that is discussed in this book, ranging from déjà vu to psychomotor, versive, grand mal, and petit mal. These experiences cannot be fully described by someone who has never had them.

As a mother of teenage daughters who may have inherited this disorder, I have a special interest in seeing that more material is published which is easy for parents, teachers, and employers to read and understand. Much of the material that is written about epilepsy is either too technical for the average person or overly simplified. In the text that follows I have tried to show the personal side of epilepsy by describing my own experiences, before examining the more technical aspects.

I have worked extensively with people in the medical profession to gain the technical understanding necessary for writing this book. F. J. L. Blasingame, M.D., of Chicago and Daniel Halpern, M.D., of Madison, Wisconsin have been especially helpful. Dr. Blasingame worked diligently with me from the inception of this section; Dr. Halpern taught me a great deal about the limbic system, while clarifying the details of cerebral palsy. Both felt, as I did, that a book about these disorders was opportune.

Thomas E. Strax, M.D., Moss Rehabilitation Center, Philadelphia, Pennsylvania; Fernando Torres, M.D., Department of Neurology at the University of Minnesota; William S. Fields, M.D., M.D. Anderson Hospital and Tumor Institute, Houston, Texas; V. Elving Anderson, Ph.D., Deight Institute, University of Minnesota; and Henri Gastaut, M.D. Medecin Chef Des Hopitaux, Neurophysiologie Clinique, Centre Hospitalier et Universitaire de Marseille, FRANCE have all been instrumental in broadening the scope of the manuscript. Joel Lubar, Ph.D., University of Tennessee, William W. Finley, M.D., of Oklahoma and B. Sterman, M.D. of the V.A. Hospital in Sepulvada, California have provided information on biofeedback.

The following pages should help to put firmly to rest the myths that have existed for years regarding epilepsy. As we say in Hawaii . . .

                                        Mahalo or Thank You,
                                        Nancy C. Schumacher

I

Seizures

A. CONVULSIVE

To consciousness, the brain is the messenger. Man
ought to know that from the brain and from the
brain only, arise the pleasures, joys, laughter and
jests, as well as our sorrow, pain, grief and tears.
Through it, in particular, we think, see, hear, and
distinguish the ugly from the beautiful, the bad
from the good, the pleasant from the unpleasant
... Hippocrates.[1]

The greek word $\epsilon\pi\iota\lambda\eta\chi\iota\alpha$,[2] which means "to seize upon"
is the basis for the word epilepsy. The disorder was recog-
nized as early as 350 B.C., when Hippocrates suggested
that the origin of epilepsy was in the brain.[3] Earlier in
history, people who suffered from convulsions were consid-

ered to be possessed by the devil or under magical power. For many years epilepsy has been, for those afflicted with it, a stigma that they could not bring themselves to accept or understand. In some cases, persons have hidden the fact when possible. They haven't told their relatives or spouses about epilepsy in their family, only to have it surface again in a later generation.

The greek word from which "epilepsy" sprung, επιληχία, suggests an aura of fear and stigma. Many misconceptions about epilepsy persist today. Some persons are afraid to associate with people with epilepsy for fear that they may be harmed in some way. They fear persons with epilepsy much as people once feared lepers.

One hundred years ago John Huglings Jackson, M.D., an English neurologist and one of the earliest to explore temporal lobe epilepsy, surmised the convulsions which he saw were evidence of brain dysfunction caused by an unruly discharge in some areas of gray matter. He was actually declaring that epilepsy has a neurophysiology of its own.[4]

Epilepsy is not a disease, it is a symptom of a neurological disorder which affects the brain. It manifests itself in the form of seizures.

The body functions on a measurable amount of electric impulses. The nervous system of an epileptic may be compared to a faulty electrical circuit. When an overload occurs, no circuit breaker is available to prevent a seizure and to keep the system running smoothly. Consequently, the ability to function is lost momentarily, in the same way that overloading an electric circuit may bring about faulty functioning.

Seizures are precipitated by chemical, physical or other irritants,[5] such as toxins, falls or certain diseases such as meningitis or encephalitis. These irritants may trigger uncontrolled firing of neurons, the nerve cells that carry electrical impulses throughout our bodies. Brain waves become quite varied during seizures, as spontaneous firing of neurons occurs.

The area of the brain in which the lesion or damage occurs affects the type of seizure which may exist. If the neural discharge remains localized, a seizure may not be observable.[6] If it spreads to regions involved in motor control, jerky, abnormal muscle contractions may occur. If the part of the brain involved with perception is affected, then hallucinatory sights, sounds, or smells may be experienced. The epileptic may feel as though he/she is progressing through a tunnel or see strange imaginary objects such as mice, chickens, or bugs. This type of seizure, however, is more of an exception.

When damage occurs to the limbic system located primarily in the temporal lobe of the brain our emotional state is effected by what are known as psychomotor seizures. Mood swings caused by such lesions may lead to behavioural problems, learning disturbances and momentary rages. Gail Solomon and Fred Plum, M.D. support this by saying: "A high incidence of behavioural disturbances, irrational behaviour, hyperactivity, schizophrenic-like personalities is found in persons with psychomotor epilepsy,"[7] but of course not every epileptic person experiences these problems.

Most simple seizures can be controlled with drugs. In cases where many areas are damaged, several types of seizures may occur simultaneously and/or at given times. This necessitates the use of more than one type of anticonvulsant. When two drugs are used to control a variety of types of seizures, one may exacerbate the type of seizure it is not designed to control.

Seizures may result from injury to the brain or temporary conditions such as concussions, digestive upsets, acute infections, or fatigue.[8] Toxins, inhalants and drugs sold on the street also sometimes bring about seizures. The onset of puberty may be another precipitating factor.

Seizures strike the person with epilepsy at any time and at any place. Stress and lack of sleep may be precipitating factors. Many people have low seizure thresholds and fight off seizures constantly. Lack of control causes them a great deal of heartache.[9] Some evidence shows that this tendency towards a low seizure threshold is often inherited.

ELECTROENCEPHALOGRAPHY

The most widely used technical aid available to physicians in diagnosing epilepsy is the electroencephalogram, called the EEG or brainwave test. The EEG is a recording of electrical activity between different points on the surface of the scalp.[10] These brainwaves are evidence of changes in voltage resulting from brain activities. The combined activities of millions of brain cells is seen in the form of wave patterns of different frequencies.

The EEG test patterns allow the physician to determine the type of seizure a person is having by discovering the location of the disturbance. This information is vital to prescribe the proper treatment. Normal EEGs are characterized by rapid, low amplitude changes in potential or voltage, evenly distributed over the entire head. The patterns shown on EEGs of people with seizure activity show more exaggerated spikes than those of normal individuals. Seizures are indicated by disruption in the rhythm of the EEG. These disruptions can occur as abnormal rhythms or as electrical discharges which are recognized on the EEG as spikes or other abnormal configurations.

The EEG test isn't any more uncomfortable than an X-ray. Electrodes are attached to the scalp to record the brain currents. The patient lies down, relaxes, and may be instructed to go to sleep. In some instances, it is necessary for the person to go into a deep sleep to get an accurate recording. In others, he/she is instructed to breathe deeply through their mouth at a rapid pace to simulate hyperventilation. This test is not always accurate, but remains one of the main tools used by the neurologist to diagnose.

The recent use of computers has advanced the art of diagnosing persons with epilepsy through the use of (Computerized Axiel Tomography) CAT scanners which use computer processing and multiple X-ray beams to produce three-dimensional images of the body. Comments William Brody of the Stanford University Medical Center, "The earliest CAT scanners narrowed the X-ray source down to a pencil-sized beam, passed it through the brain in one plane from every possible direction, then put the information into a computer. And the computer, lo and behold, can construct a picture of the plane. It essentially saws the brain in two. The first scanner 12 years ago took 15 minutes to collect the information and 12 hours to reconstruct the image. Now scanners with multiple X-ray beams routinely acquire the same data in one second and reconstruct the image in thirty."[11] This test has become most effective in determining if a person does have a tumor, rather than epilepsy.

One of the new and experimental devices is the Positron Emission Tomograph (PET Scan) which penetrates the human body's metabolism by recording traces of "nuclear annihilation" in body tissue.

Jack Fincher[12] describes the PET scanner as follows:

> "A patient receives short-lived radioactive tracers, combined with chemicals the body normally uses. The tracers emit particles called "positrons" that collide with electrons less than a few millimeters away, and produce bursts of energy that detectors record. As these collisions continue repeatedly, the detectors slowly build up a map of just where the tracer chemical is or is not being metabolized. The tracers can be chemically custom tailored to measure blood flow and volume, oxygen and protein metabolism and other factions.
>
> Although it is still an experimental device the PET scanner is already being used clinically to test for Alzheimer's disease (a form of progressive degeneration of the brain), to locate the malfunctioning part of an epileptic's brain, and to evaluate a stroke's effects."

As mechanization increases the physician's ability to see into the brain, it will become possible to accurately diagnose the problems which lie there.

*   *   *

CLASSIFICATION

Epileptic seizures are classified in four types: grand mal, major or generalized seizures; petit mal or absence seizures; minor motor attacks; focal seizures-motor, sensory and psychomotor attacks.

Scientists use various names for the four types of seizures. In the following discussion, the old terminology is used—grand mal, petit mal, minor motor seizures and focal seizures—because it is more frequently used.

TABLE 1

OLD AND NEW TERMINOLOGY FOR SEIZURES[13]

Grand mal	generalized-tonic-clonic
Petit mal	generalized-absence
Focal Motor or sensory seizures	focal and partial, simple or elementary symptomatology focal and partial, complex.
idiopathic	unclassified

Grand Mal

Grand mal seizures, or generalized convulsions, are usually considered the most common type of seizure. They occur in approximately 90 percent of patients, either alone or in combination with other forms. It usually lasts five minutes or more in the rigid convulsive (tonic-clonic) stages. Such an attack may be preceded by an epileptic cry and an aura or warning in the form of an unusual sensory experience.

The convulsion encompasses the entire body. Strong muscular contractions occur during which the body becomes rigid. These contractions are called tonic contractions, or the tonic phase. During this phase, the body may be held so rigidly that breathing is interfered with and a patient's skin may turn blue. This phase is usually followed by a clonic phase in which back, arm, and leg muscles contract alternatingly. During the seizure the person salivates profusely, breathing speeds up and slows down and eyes roll upwards. Loss of bladder control is also common during this generalized seizure.

The clonic phase is followed by a deep coma or post-seizure (ictal) state, from which the person may not easily be aroused. If a grand mal seizure is very intense, the person may have difficulty speaking or writing when he comes out of the post-seizure state. In any case, a terrible headache can be expected on awakening. On rare occasions, recall may be delayed for several days.

The frequency and severity of these attacks vary dramatically. Episodes may last for less than a minute or over ten minutes. These episodes can occur several times a day or only once in several years. The attacks may be predominantly nocturnal, occuring in sleep, but are usually spread throughout the entire twenty-four hours. The person may be aware of the attacks or, if they occur during sleep, may be completely unaware of the form they take. In some cases they may recall strange hallucinations. These seizures have been known to keep people in limbo for as long as forty-one hours, with the effects not wearing off completely for sixty-five hours (in which case they can be considered non-convulsive status).[14] Complete recall may not return for several days, but such severe attacks are rare.

Petit Mal

Petit mal seizures are a second type of generalized seizure. They are often referred to as absence seizures, because the patient appears to be out of contact with his surroundings for the five to thirty seconds. Petit mal seizures are more common in childhood and rarely begin in adulthood. Two to five percent of epileptics suffer from petit mal seizures— about 48,500 people.[15] Of these only about 25 per cent become seizure free by age twenty, 50 percent develop grand mal epilepsy.

This type of seizure may sometimes go undetected. A teacher may think that the child who stares intently for short periods of time is merely inattentive or daydreaming. If these seizures are too numerous, however, a child may have difficulty concentrating on school work. The child who has petit mal may also appear disobedient because he/she does not hear the teacher or parent. The child may experience the world as flashing on and off, like a TV set.

Minor Motor

Minor motor seizures may be characterized by sudden loss of movement and falling episodes where muscle activities are suddenly interrupted. The first type may be called *akinetic*, meaning sudden loss of movement, because individuals suddenly drop to the ground. The second type, *myoclonic jerks*, are sudden involuntary muscular contractions of the trunk and limbs. These somewhat resemble petit mal in that they are very brief, frequent and asymetric. The arms and chest may be propelled forward in a jackknife position, or the head may merely nod. The episodes last about a second, usually with no loss of consciousness.[16]

The third type of minor motor seizures, *infantile spasms*, may take the form of massive myoclonic episodes. These usually occur in infants many times a day and tend to be associated with brain damage and mental retardation. This syndrome, known as West's syndrome, is often confused with tics, colic, or abdominal difficulty.[17]

Focal

As opposed to minor motor seizures, focal seizures may be characterized by movement, sensory phenomena such as strange sounds or smell, or a combination of the two.

1. One form, *automatic seizures*, affects the automatic nervous system, which is comprised of all the efferent nerves (carrying impulses away from a nerve center) through which the organs of the heart, glands and peripheral involuntary muscles are innervated.[18] Seizures may remain localized in a single part of the body or progress to a generalized form with loss of consciousness. Focal seizures may be followed by periods of immobility of the affected limbs.[19]

2. A *Motor seizure* is a type of focal seizure which

occurs when electrical discharge in one part of the brain extends into the section which controls motor activity.[20] *Jacksonian, versive* and *aphasic seizures* are the three types of motor seizures most commonly seen.

a. *Jacksonian epilepsy* involves recurrent muscle contractions in the same muscle group. Beginning in the thumb or toe, they spread over the muscles on one side of the body,[21] and may or may not culminate in a generalized seizure accompanied by the loss of consciousness. If the left portion of the brain is affected speech may be lost momentarily.[22]

b. *Versive seizures* are characterized by the head and eyes being drawn away from the affected area. As the head and eyes turn to the side, and the hand and arm extend, a circling movement begins.[23] Consciousness may be lost as the person circles, trips and falls.[24] Speech is also affected.

c. *Aphasic seizures* arise through damage to the speech area (Broca's area) of the brain. Broca (1861) discovered that lesions destroying the lower section of the frontal lobe result in the inability to formulate the words necessary for speech. Because this difficulty represents a coordination of the motor activities required for speech, it has been called *motor aphasia*.

Brief stereotyped utterences (speech automatism) may occur with damage to the temporal lobes of either side of the brain.[25] Damage to a portion of the parietal lobe on the left side of the brain interferes with the ability to associate words with the objects or ideas they represent. This impairment results in a deficiency in the ability to use language as a process for symbolizing thoughts.[26]

Either or both difficulties in carrying out motor activities or using language may be evident during the course of a seizure. Seizures causing aphasic reactions can be likened to nervous storms which momentarily interrupt the ability to formulate words, speak coherently, or to understand the speech of others. Grave difficulties may arise if the person is not among people who are aware of his condition.

3. *Sensory seizures,* during which a person may see, hear, feel or taste (unusual and different things) are another form of focal seizures.

4. *Complex partial seizures* incorporate many of the symptoms of focal seizures already described above. They are especially frequent in persons suffering from temporal lobe epilepsy. Profound disturbances of thought, perception, emotions and behaviour may be experienced during the seizure.[27]

The phenomena of *déjà vu* and *jamais vu* are typical expressions of complex partial seizures. The person may have an overwhelming sense that a given situation has occurred before (déjà-vu).[28,29] Or a person may perceive familiar surroundings as unfamiliar and disorienting (jamais vu). For example: a person suffering from this form of sensory seizure may stand at a bus stop where he/she has caught the bus daily for the past twenty years without recognizing their surroundings. Or even in their own home with their own family they may still have no idea who they are or why they are there. Another phenomenon of complex partial seizures is *forced thinking.* This occurs when the affected person has an ungrounded fear (such as a fear of being strangled), or experiences a recurrent hallucination during the onset of each seizure.[30]

The *psychomotor seizure* is a type of complex partial

seizure. It may incorporate any or all of the above phenomena and occurs in people with temporal lobe lesions. Those who experience psychomotor seizures lose consciousness for a few seconds to fifteen minutes or longer. These episodes may occur off and on for several days. The person's behaviour is often altered and he/she may say and do things that they would not ordinarily do. Fumbling with clothes, talking senselessly, putting the butter in the oven instead of the refrigerator are typical examples of how the epileptic can be totally confused and disoriented. Police have mistakenly arrested such persons during these seizures, believing them to be intoxicated.

Some researchers are of the opinion that more than fifty percent of epileptics belong to this type.[31] It is known to be one of the most common epileptic disorders of children, accounting for 35–45 percent of the cases investigated in recent years.[32] The three subgroups of psychomotor seizures are found in the following proportions: 37%-automatic, 25%-subjective, tonic and focal features, 30%-arrest of motion and mentation.[33] Loss of recall may also be affected.

*　　　　　*　　　　　*

It is important to distinguish between seizures which are the symptoms of epilepsy and the disorder which is recognized by a continuous reoccurence of seizures. The location of the lesion may affect the individuals' mood; their control over their depression, their anger and their ability to control fear.[34] Recent literature has questioned whether these emotions are the result or the cause of seizures.[35,36,37] It has long been known that emotions can be a part of the aura.

Fear as an experience occurs only when the lesion discharge involves the anterior half of the temporal lobe. If the central core area of the brain, known as the limbic system is closely affected by lesions, anger or depression may occur in the person's behaviour. Complex epileptic experiences result from lesions or discharges in many parts of the brain. Fear arises in 70 percent of the 50 patients with anterior temporal lesions, and in 46 percent of the 47 with middle temporal lesions and in 60 percent of both groups.[38]

HANDLING A SEIZURE

It is important to know how to handle a person during a seizure. Such knowledge prevents panic and enables one to take the appropriate action quickly. Many myths regarding the proper management of a seizure remain, such as placing something in the person's mouth to prevent him from swallowing his tongue. No such danger exists because of the structure of the tongue; indeed, foreign objects forced into the mouth may result in strangulation or injury to the teeth and soft mouth structures.

The Epilepsy Foundation of America suggests the following guidelines:

1. *Keep calm* when a major seizure occurs. You cannot stop a seizure once it has started. Do not restrain the patient or try to revive them.
2. *Clear the area* around them of hard, sharp or hot objects which could injure them. Place a pillow or rolled-up mat under their head.
3. *Do not force anything between the teeth.* If their

mouth is open, you might place a soft object like a handkerchief between the side teeth.

4. *Turn the patient's head to the side*, and make sure their breathing is not obstructed. Loosen necktie and tight clothing but do not interfere with their movements.

5. *Do not be concerned* if they seem to stop breathing momentarily. *Do be concerned* if they begin to pass from one seizure into another without gaining consciousness. This is rare but requires a doctor's help.

6. *Carefully observe the patient's actions* during the seizures for a full medical report later. When the seizure is over the patient should rest if they wish.[39]

These suggestions are merely an outline of the ground rules; the more you know about epilepsy, the easier it is to deal with seizures in a helpful manner.

*   *   *

B. NON-CONVULSIVE

Et tú Brutè

Marcia gave a sigh of relief as she closed the book, *Nerves in Collision*. Although she could not agree with everything in Dr. Walter Alverez's book, it was reassuring to know that other people had problems similar to her own.

For the past fifteen years she had been married to a wonderful man, a good worker who did not smoke or drink, and who participated in family life. Roger enjoyed people and had a lot of friends. During the time he had spent in the service, he had received several honorable character awards.

Yet, this same man, usually so understanding and helpful, could be unreasonably angry if he felt that his word was being questioned. Many times his anger had caused him to become quite violent with Marcia. She had decided years ago that he did not realize just how strong he was when he became enraged. For many years, Roger had had trouble with tinnitus . . . or a ringing in his ears. This of course, made him edgy. Even so, she found it difficult to understand and accept his actions.

Then something happened that helped to explain Roger's mood swings. He began having grand mal seizures in his sleep. They would usually begin about 3 a.m. and last approximately five minutes. Marcia recognized grand mal seizures because she had epilepsy herself. Her ability to recognize the seizure for what it was did not lessen the intense fear which she felt. When the seizures occurred, she followed the directions given by the Epilepsy Foundation of America. She tried to keep calm, wiped the saliva from his mouth, and carefully turned his head so that he would not choke. After the tonic-clonic portion of the seizure had ceased, he sank into a deep sleep.

The following morning, Roger did not remember anything. He did have a headache. And the ringing in his ears was back again, more intense than usual. When Marcia told him what had happened, he could not believe that he had actually had a seizure. However, he did feel very tired. His muscles ached and his head pounded. At his wife's insistence he made an appointment with a neurologist. The next day he returned to work and tried to ignore the event.

At eleven day intervals, for the next two months he had a similar seizure at the same hour in the early morning. After negative results from a routine EEG and a CAT scan, the neurologist finally got some irregular readings from a sleep EEG. He placed Roger on Dilantin three times daily. When his seizures ceased, Roger tried to convince his wife that he no longer had a problem and tried taking less medication. This proved to be a serious mistake and his seizures returned.

When he had been a teenager Roger had had some blackouts and one doctor even had mentioned the word "epilepsy". His father had taken him to a chiropractor, however, and the attacks had stopped. He joined the Army, spent thirty-one years in service to his country and really enjoyed military life. He had worked with delicate machinery which necessitated intricate movements and an alert mind. Today he held a place of considerable responsibility in his company. During all this time Roger had assumed that the only problem had been a "jarred nerve" . . . apparently jarred back into place by the chiropractor. At age forty-six, it was extremely difficult to think of himself as a possible epileptic even though epilepsy was a part of his wife's life.

Marcia suffered from a complex form of seizures which had never been under complete control. When he married her, Roger had told her flatly that he would never let her drive because it simply was not safe. Now the idea of having to live under similar restrictions was very upsetting. He simply would not believe it. Why should he take the Dilantin which had been prescribed? He did not have the problems. Perhaps he got upset sometimes, but everyone got upset under certain circumstances. When his wife showed him the book about significant signs of non-convulsive epileptics, he refused to read it.

*   *   *

PSYCHO-SOCIAL ASPECTS

Epilepsy is a physical condition, but also inevitably affects all other aspects of one's life. Successful treatment of a person with epilepsy cannot be accomplished without considering the entire individual. In the past, the psycho-social aspects of epilepsy have often been overlooked or not given the importance due them, and this may cause more damage than the seizures themselves.

Epilepsy is viewed with a great deal of fear and misunderstanding by most people. To many people, the word epilepsy conjures up a picture of someone falling, writhing and lying unconscious. This view focusses attention on the disability in an exaggerated manner and can prevent acceptance of the individual as a person. There are many different forms of epilepsy. For this reason, it is much less accepted or understood than diabetes, another chronic disorder. Many people with epilepsy are rejected by their peers and relatives. Consequently, life in our society may seem threatening and unfair until the individual with epilepsy can learn to cope with these problems. He/she may tend to grow very angry or ashamed and accuse others of failing to understand their circumstances, and thus create an intolerable situation.

Writing in 1904, W. P. Spratling observed that persons

with epilepsy could be detected because of the "ill-humor periods" which precede the onset of seizures. He estimated such temperamental changes to occur in up to 80 percent of persons with seizures.[40] Uncontrollable changes in mood are another important part of the psychosocial makeup of the individual.

Because of the significant psychological features of the disorder, there is an urgent need for programs to educate the public—especially teachers—and to assist the epileptic whose problems in finding help and developing better skills for coping seem insurmountable.

Since epilepsy often begins in childhood, parents must also be educated. People who have grown up with an antipathy towards epilepsy will inevitably look at this disorder as a catastrophe for their child, and may find it difficult to accept that their child is not perfect, or is "deficient" in some manner. They can learn to deal with it by accepting the conditions or by denying its existence and rejecting the child who suffers the consequences of the disorder.

Even parents who try to deal with the problems may not initially understand its consequences. They may become overprotective, which often has a negative effect on the child. As a consequence of not having to take care of his or her needs, the overprotected child is typically passive and yet quite demanding. Much of the time, they may be selfish and often less willing to express their actions and ideas with others. On the other hand, people who are trained to develop friendships and depend on themselves usually find it easier to get along in the world. Parents who appreciate that there is a great deal of hostility in the world may unwittingly place an unnecessary burden on their child through overprotectiveness. Parents become properly supportive only when they teach their children the skills which help them to deal with society's reactions to their disability.

Society does not make life easy for those with disabilities. The stigma associated with epilepsy may cause some parents to feel that they must keep their child's defect a secret. Without fully realizing the consequences of their actions, they are asking their child to live the life of an unaffected person and still be themselves. This creates a tension which is difficult for the child to understand and only compounds the problem of coping with the disorder. The person with epilepsy who has been brought up in an overprotected environment suffers a double shock when he or she enters real-life situations. This in turn aggravates the psychological problems which the individual may have. If the seizures are well controlled, others may not be aware that there is a problem, but the individual who is told to hide a seizure condition must always live with the fear of the secret being discovered. This threat in itself causes unwarranted anxiety and stress which may itself be likely to cause seizures.

Those parents who seek to avoid the reality of their child's disorder may avoid admitting to themselves or their child that there actually is a problem. They may fail to tell the child why the medication is necessary or fail to administer it at all. In one such case, the parents told their young child, who was taking Dilantin, that the drug was administered for a stomach disorder. In high school, when he was suddenly confronted with the real reason for the drug being administered, he had to undergo a much more difficult period of readjustment. By rejecting the child and/or the disorder parents inevitably find themselves dealing with an insecure child—and sometimes even an emotionally disturbed one.

By the time they are old enough for school, many children with epilepsy may have psychological in addition to physical problems. They often have difficulty achieving the scholastic performance of which they are capable. It is important for teachers to know and understand that a child has epilepsy and to be conscious of its implications.

For those children who have seizures during class, it is important for the staff to understand the disorder and be able to cope with the problems that arise. As many as ⅔ of preschool children show some hyperactivity due to psychomotor epilepsy.[41] One-fourth of children with psychomotor epilepsy show signs of hyperactivity.[42] For these children the inability to concentrate may be a significant problem. They may be thought of as not paying attention and constantly daydreaming, when they are actually having petit mal seizures. They may appear overly hyperactive or only inattentive. Adolescent epileptics may misbehave or even find themselves in serious trouble with the law in an attempt to escape from rejection or overprotection. In some older children with temporal lobe epilepsy a particular type of behaviour develops. They become slow, circumstantial and perseverative in their speech, move on to other topics with great difficulty and dislike interruptions. They are persistent, pedantic and "sticky" in their motor and contact behaviour.[43]

Some people have more difficulty handling their anger than others. Those with damage to the frontal lobe or limbic system (principally in the temporal lobe) find it more difficult to control their anger than nonaffected people.

Self-discipline is needed to handle other frustrations as well. For example, they may have difficulty accepting the fact that a person who has affronted them really did not mean to.

When caught in a stress-filled situation in family living, or a situation which continues to engender criticism or insensitivity, the person with epilepsy (especially the person with limbic damage) is susceptible to an avalanche of seizures which cannot always be completely controlled by drugs.

The spouse of the person with epilepsy may not realize his or her ability to prevent or precipitate stressful situations. If the spouse does not comprehend the importance of this position, something may be said or done which causes the epileptic unnecessary pain. For most people with epilepsy it is important to be able to talk about the seizures when they occur in such a way that their importance is not blown out of proportion. Talking things over can assist the person with epilepsy in being realistic about a problem which must be faced.

Kind and considerate handling of the epileptic during a seizure is extremely important. In one case, an agitated wife slapped the face of her epileptic husband in order to bring him around. Unfortunately, this only served to antagonize him. He was conscious but unable to speak. No doubt the spouse meant well, but understanding was sorely lacking.

Persons with epilepsy often refrain from marrying because they feel inferior, incapable or likely to be misunderstood. Overprotection by parents seems to influence the making of such a decision negatively. When it has been difficult for a person to make and maintain friends earlier in life, it stands to reason that it may be even more difficult later to find someone who will be a good partner for life. Parents who start early to teach their children to get along with others show wisdom and understanding and help the children to learn to cope with life.

Many epileptics lead normal lives and their seizures are either completely or partially controlled by medication. Others have problems. The more difficult it is to control seizures with medication, the more likely the person is to have trouble holding a job and coping socially or psychologically.

The fears which persons with epilepsy experience are commonplace to all people, but in epileptics they may become blown out of proportion. Especially upsetting is the feeling that they may become more and more dependent on others.

Persons who have a great deal of hardship controlling their seizures are seen in rehabilitation centers and in the Comprehensive Epilepsy Programs. In these programs testing is done to obtain a better perspective on the epileptic's personality traits, as well as to ascertain if there has been any brain damage. Minimal brain damage may affect a person by interfering with decision-making and an ability to plan and adapt to life.[44]

The Comprehensive Epilepsy Program works with individuals to obtain a psycho-social evaluation in terms of family, job, self, and interpersonal relationships. All this promotes activities which will assist in the development of coping skills and the ability to interact within the community. Teams of nurses, doctors, social workers and psychologists are available to meet the individual's needs. Occupational therapists evaluate work skills in vocational counseling.

Social workers, psychologists and neurologists provide family counseling. Major problems of developing friendships and controlling anger are also dealt with. Obviously, the physician's first responsibility is to try to achieve seizure control, but complete control of seizures is ineffective if the individual remains frustrated and impeded by an inability to control anger, hold a job and relate to others.

A treatment program such as the Comprehensive Epilepsy Program works when both the individual and the members of the team work together honestly reporting the occurrence of seizures and medications administered. The Program has been established in many hospitals throughout the country. It deals with living in the real world and is made as "non-hospitalized" as possible in order to treat the whole person.

Since epilepsy can strike people at different ages, the time when the disorder begins will also affect the way a person handles the disorder. The teenager who has not been able to obtain a driver's license will have great difficulty accepting the fact. They are likely to feel antagonism toward themselves and their disorder. The inability to drive marks them as someone who is not "in".

Adults over fifty years old, suddenly stricken with the disorder, must change their lifestyles. In some cases, it means that they must change occupations. The adult may have difficulty accepting the change and, consequently, may feel it unlikely that their family can accept them. Most mid-career epileptics must cope with a great deal of anxiety and frustration.

The child who grows up with epilepsy in an accepting household learns at an early age to accept it. They treat it as an integral part of their personality that cannot be forced to go away. Those children who are overprotected or rejected will be more likely to reject their disorder and magnify the problem. There are no two exact situations. Each is unique and must be dealt with on an individual basis.

*   *   *

II

Treatments

In order for people to seek treatment, they must be adequately motivated to do so. Unfortunately, a high percentage of epileptics do not see physicians at all, and over 5 percent never see a specialist.[45] A patient may be reluctant to see a doctor when he/she rarely has seizures. They may feel that it is only a temporary problem which will go away. If seizures occur during their sleep, they may not be aware of them, consequently they believe there is no reason to seek assistance. Other people become "addicted", as it were, to their attacks. They feel that they can control other people by the frequency of their attacks. Although they do not enjoy them, they do enjoy the attention which they receive. Still other people actually enjoy the feelings which the aura provides.[46] Support groups and individual help may enable them to see the fallacy in both situations.

Cases in which the patient has had little or no help from the treatment and has become spoiled or "molly-coddled" by others are less common.[47] These people do not wish to give up their way of life. They lack the incentive to seek and follow treatment so may resist drug therapy which might prevent their seizure activity. Personalized attention is needed to direct these people toward support programs which can enable them to live more meaningful lives.

DRUG THERAPY continues to be the method used most for controlling seizures. Some patients suffer from mixed varieties of seizures and are more difficult to treat with drugs. A drug which will control petit mal may aggravate grand mal seizures and vice-versa. Various drugs produce feelings of euphoria or depression in some individuals. Consequently, physicians often must juggle the medication to match the needs of the patient.

Drugs are used not only to control seizures but to save lives as well. In status epilepticus the person goes from one seizure into another without regaining consciousness. An ordinary epileptic convulsion is followed by a period during which the person is exhausted. In status epilepticus, on the other hand, the mechanism of exhaustion fails.[48] One seizure follows another without an intermittent lull. This situation may occur with any type of seizure. Such a series of seizures is life threatening. Immediate treatment is necessary and essential. Drugs must be injected directly into the veins to counter continuing attacks (See p. 69).

SURGERY today, more than at any time in the past, is successfully being performed on patients with lesions. Unfortunately, not everyone is a candidate for surgery. The lesions must be in a specific place for it to be successful;[49] and even this concept is controversial.

NUTRITION is also used today to treat epilepsy. Through the efforts of a new school of physicians, known as doctors of "orthomolecular medicine", more importance is being placed on the aspects of metabiology and nutrition.

BIOFEEDBACK is another form of treatment which is just beginning to be taken seriously as a tool in fighting epilepsy. Individuals learn to treat themselves as they systematically observe their own actions and reactions and are taught to relax in order to control their own seizures without medication . . . or with only a portion of the medication upon which they once depended.

GENETIC COUNSELING is used to enable people to assess the possibility that they may carry the disorder onto their children. Certain types of seizures have a genetic component and it is felt by some geneticists that epilepsy can be hereditary.[50]

*   *   *

A. Drugs

One of the most successful ways of treating epilepsy is through the use of anticonvulsants and stimulants in drug therapy. Some drugs are more effective with specific types of seizure disorders than are others.

Today, a wide selection of drugs is available to patients. Anti-epileptic drugs may inhibit the discharge of abnormal neurons or prevent the spread of the discharge once it has begun.[51] A combination of these effects is also possible.[52]

As early as 1847 bromides proved effective as the first anti-epileptic drug when Sir Charles Locock used potassium bromide to treat the disorder.[53] Today, there are four basic divisions of anticonvulsants: barbiturates, hydantoins, oxozoladines, and succinimides.[54] The following is a short discussion of anti-convulsants that have been used most effectively to control seizure activity. According to reports, the usage of these drugs seems to vary with regions of the country.

Barbiturates

The most commonly used barbiturates are phenobarbital (Luminal); mephobarbital (Meberal); and metharbital (Gemonil).[55] Phenobarbital was introduced in 1912 and has remained one of the most widely used anti-epileptic drugs to date. Known in Europe as Luminal, it can cause dullness and drowsiness, mild dysarthria (difficulty in articulation of speech) and nystagmus (involuntary rapid movement of the eyeball) when taken in large dosages.[56]

A low dosage of phenobarbital relieves mild or moderate anxiety. Higher dosage taken at bedtime induces sleep. Phenobarbital acts on the connecting points of synapses in the nerve pathways that transmit impulses from the wake-sleep areas of the brain.[57] This is not as simple as it sounds and is not yet fully understood.

Mephobarbital (Meberal) works in a similar manner, and there is no clear evidence about which is more effective.[58] Mephobarbital is used as a sedative to relieve anxiety, tension and apprehension, as well as to control grand mal seizures. It can be used along with phenytoin (Dilantin). Status epilepticus may result from abrupt withdrawal of this medication.[59]

Metharbital (Gemonil) is a synthetic derivative of phenobarbital. It is similar in effect as those produced by phenobartital and mephobarbital. It is sometimes used for the control of grand mal, petit mal, myoclonic and mixed types of seizures.[60,61] Since the drug is detoxified primarily in the liver, it should be used with caution by persons with liver conditions. Side effects include rashes, dizziness, gastric disorders and increased irritability.[62] The mechanisms by which these drugs work are not fully understood.

Hydantoins

Hydantoins available today are diphenylhydantoin sodium (Dilantin or phenytoin), mephenytoin (Messantoin) and ethotoin (Peganone). Dilantin seems to be considered the most effective hydantoin used currently for the management of major grand mal and psychomotor epilepsy. It was introduced in 1938. Researchers believe that Dilantin promotes loss of sodium from nerve cells, which lowers and stabilizes their excitability and inhibits the repetitious spread of electrical impulses along nerve pathways.[63] This action may prevent seizures altogether or may at least reduce their frequency. It may, however, have adverse effects on the central nervous system. The most common side effect is a functional disturbance of the cerebellar connections of the brainstem,[64] producing course nystagmus or lateral gaze, ataxia (difficulty in coordinating voluntary muscles) and slurred speech.

Changes of mood and movements (inadvertent flexing and extension of muscles) may also occur.[65, 66] Other side effects include overgrowth of gums (gingival hyperplasia), excessive growth of hair, especially in women (hirsutism) and a decrease in white blood cells (megablastic anemia and leucopenia). Dilantin is metabolized chiefly by the liver where it may become highly concentrated. Patients with liver impairment may show early toxicity.[67]

Of more recent origin is methylphenylhydantoin (Mesantoin) which has been a very active anti-epileptic drug, but not without some undesirable side effects. It has been known to cause aplastic anemia, ataxia, skin rash and drowsiness.

Ethotoin (Peganone) is a hydantoin derivative which acts similarly to Dilantin in the body in that the drug acts to stabilize the normal threshold rather than raise it. The grand mal and psychomotor seizures are the most effectively controlled by this action. Persons who take the drug are advised to make certain that their blood level is checked on a regular basis. Although ethotoin is relatively free of swollen gums and hirsutism,[68] side effects such as fatigue, insomnia, dizziness, headache, diplopia (double vision), nystagmus, rash, and chest pains do occur.[69] Ataxia is rare.[70]

Oxozoladines

The oxozoladine used most today is trimethadione (Tridione). This drug was introduced in 1945 and has worked quite well in relieving petit mal conditions. Unfortunately, it can give rise to toxins in the blood, which makes frequent examination of blood levels necessary.[71] Another side effect is photophobia, which causes the person to see hallucinatory colored objects and brings about a temporary disturbance in color vision.[72]

Succinimides

Succinimides in existence today are ethnosuximide (Zarontin), phenosuximide (Milontin) and methosuximide (Celontin). Ethnosuximide (Zarontin) was developed in 1960. It may be used instead of trimethadione[73] to control petit mal seizures. Blood level checks must be maintained. This drug may leave a person with a feeling of euphoria. It may also affect the ability to use the muscles of the hands. It is effective mainly with petit mal, and ineffective on grand mal or psychomotor seizures. This drug is sometimes administered with other drugs to people having a combination of types of epilepsy. Leukopenia, a loss of white blood cells, and a dangerous form of anemia is the major side effect.[74]

Phenosuximide (Milontin) was introduced in 1953. It is also used only for petit mal seizures. It elevates the threshold of neurons in order to inhibit the excitation of nerve cells in the body.

Methosuximide (Celontin) was introduced in 1957.[75] It was used to control temporal lobe epilepsy in conjunction with other drugs. Leukopenia may occur as a side effect.

*   *   *

The following anti-convulsants do not fall into the above mentioned groups. They are important anti-epileptic drugs in their own right.

Carbamazepine (Tegretol) was used in Europe as an anti-convulsant long before it was approved in the United States, where it was used as a therapeutic agent for trigeminal neuralgia. Today, it is approved as an anti-convulsant. It is useful in the treatment of generalized tonic-clonic seizures, but is even more effective in the treatment of psychomotor (complex partial) and mixed seizure patterns.[76, 77] It has no effect on petit mal.

Side effects include vertigo, ataxia, diplopia (double vision) and drowsiness. The blood count of patients on this drug should be monitored regularly. It should be withdrawn immediately if bone marrow suppression occurs. Persons having difficulty with adverse blood reactions are at risk under this drug.[78, 79] It is recommended for persons whose seizures are very difficult to control.

In 1960 primidone (Mysoline) desoxyphenylethlmalonylurea was introduced. It has proven to be distinctly helpful in treating grand mal, psychomotor and focal seizures which fail to respond to other drugs.[80] A combination of phenobarbital and phenylethlmalonamide (PMMA),[81] primidone raises electro-chemoshock seizure threshold or alters seizure patterns,[82] and may be combined effectively with phenytoin or mephenytoin.[83] If toxic effects occur, they usually do so within the first few days and tend to decrease with use. Primidone may cause some people to be irritable.[84] Although some people may be hypersensitive to this drug, it is frequently used by many physicians. Adverse effects include ataxia and vertigo. Nausea, anoxia, fatigue, hyperirritability, emotional disturbances, impotence, diplopia and megablastic anemia have also been reported.[85] Primidone reduces and stabilizes the excitability of nerve fibers and inhibits the repetitious spread of electrical impulses along nerve pathways. This may prevent seizures altogether or it may reduce their frequency and severity. Part of this drug's action is attributed to phenobarbital, one of its conversion products in the body.[86]

Clonazepam (Clonopin) is used to prevent some petit mal or absence seizures. There is also increasing evidence of its effectiveness in treating psychomotor (complex partial) seizures. It is not yet FDA approved for this condition however, because its mechanism of action is unknown.[87] Side effects are common and include ataxia, drowsiness, and occasional behavior disorders in children. Very gradual increases in dosage is suggested.

Diazepam (Valium) is used exclusively as a tranquilizer but has demonstrated definite anti-convulsive activities in experimental animals.[88] Benzodiazepines were broadly used by neurologists after H. Gastaut released a report of several cases of status epilepticus treatment with diazepam.[89]

It is considered, by some experts in the United States, the drug of choice for control of this type of seizure; it may be used intravaneously to correct this condition.[90] Toxic effects include drowsiness, constipation, diplopia, headache, hypertension, rash, and slurred speech.[91]

Lorazepam, a benzodiazepine with potent anti-convulsant activity in animal models,[92] may be effective for treatment of status epilepticus. A double-blind study released in the March, 1982 issue of JAMA by Ilo E. Leppik, M.D., et. al., gives a comparison of the two benzodiazepines—lorazepam and diazepam. This study compares their immediate effectiveness, time of onset of action and adverse side effects in a random study of seventy-eight patients. Earlier studies of the drug have indicated that it has a longer duration of anti-convulsant activity than diazepam.[93] Although more clinical experience is needed, it is felt that this drug will act more effectively than phenytoin or diazepam to quickly control status epilepticus. Results from this study indicate that lorazepam is at least as effective as diazepam in the initial treatment of status.[94] People accepted for the study included those having grand mal, absence and partial elementary and partial complex seizures. Respiratory arrest seemed to be the main adverse reaction.

Sodium valproate (Depakane) is chemically unrelated to the other drugs that are used to treat seizure disorders as it is a short-chain fatty acid. The mechanism by which the drug exerts its effects is unknown. Sodium valproate was first synthesized in 1881, and used as a solvent to disolve other compounds. In 1963 French investigators discovered that compounds which had been disolved in sodium valproate acted to prevent seizures in mice.

Eighty-two years after it was synthesized, sodium valproate was investigated for its anti-epileptic properties. In 1964, the first clinical trials of the drug were reported in a French medical journal. It has been used in Europe since that time, but was not approved in the United States until 1978. Adverse side effects include transient hair loss, skin rash, ataxia, headache, nausea, nystagmus, tremor, dysarthria, dizziness and weight gain.[95, 96] Since this drug is relatively new to the United States, it has not been tested as thoroughly as others. However, it offers some hope to those who have not yet found a drug which works. It is most effective with absence, myoclonic, tonic-clonic and mixed absence seizures.[97] It has been known to cause people to see colors and, like any anti-convulsant, it should not be withdrawn abruptly without expecting seizure recurrence to result.

Stimulants

Methylphenidate (Ritalin) was developed in 1956 and was first used for hyperactive children in 1958. At one time it was used with adult epileptics as a stimulant to offset some of the effects of anti-convulsants, but this is done less frequently today.

Ritalin improves a person's confidence, initiative and performance. It is believed that the drug acts by increasing the release of the nerve impulse transmitter, norepinephrine. The resulting stimulation of the brain tissue improves alertness and concentration and increases learning ability and attention span.[98]

Amphetamines were used in treatment of hyperactivity more than thirty years ago when Bradley discovered their paradoxical calming effects on hyperactive patients. Since then virtually every psychopharmacological agent has been tested on children who have minimal brain damage. Unfortunately, controlled studies are limited and reports conflict as to the type of child likely to respond favorably.[99]

*   *   *

STATUS EPILEPTICUS AND DRUG THERAPY

As stated earlier in the chapter, status epilepticus, or the condition in which a person goes from one seizure into another without regaining consciousness, can be brought about by failure to take medications and/or by reducing medication too quickly. An ordinary seizure is followed by a period during which the person is exhausted and the seizure stops.[100] Status epilepticus can be very dangerous without immediate treatment. Phenytoin is the drug most often used. In some instances, diazepam has been preferred. Either drug may be administered directly into the veins by a health care professional. In future years, lorazepam may be used instead.

*   *   *

There is a distinct need for new improved, safer and more effective drugs. Pharmacists and physicians are constantly trying to discover safer and more effective drugs, but each new drug involves unforseen risks, and it is sometimes difficult to remain optomistic.

As indicated earlier, for medication to be successful it must be suited to the individual. Anti-convulsants are carefully monitored so that the physician in charge is aware of the blood's white, red and platelet count. White blood cells fight off infection; red cells carry oxygen and platelets promote blood clotting. An allergic reaction may prevent production of any of these elements in the bone marrow and lead to anemia or leukopenia. Such a reaction may affect the cells as they circulate in the bloodstream, causing them to stick together and disintegrate.

TABLE 2

TREATMENT OF SPECIFIC TYPES OF EPILEPSY

Seizure type	First Choice	Second Choice	Other Drugs
Generalized tonic-clonic seizures	Diphenylhydantoin	Carbamazepine	Phenobarbital primidone, sodium valproate
Generalized tonic seizures	As above	As above	As above
Generalized clonic seizures	As above	As above	As above
Myoclonus epilepsy	As above	As above	As above
Secondary generalized seizures	As above	As above	Clonazepam
Infantile spasm	ACTH	Carbamazepine	Clonazepam diphenylhydantoin, Phenobarbital
Absence	Ethnosuximide	Sodium Valproate	Clonazepam
Atypical absence			
Akinetic seizures	Ethosuximide	Clonazepam	
Continuing absence	IV diazepam		
Partial seizures with complex symptomatology	Diphenylhydantoin	Carbamazepine	Primidone, sodium valproate, clonazepam

Gilroy, John, M.D. and Meyer, John Stirling, M.D. MEDICAL NEUROLOGY 1969 Macmillan Publishing Co., p. 365.

The side effects of any drug must be weighed against its ability to control seizures. Drugs must be prescribed to increase a person's overall ability to lead a normal life. When toxicity occurs drugs must be changed, and sometimes dosage must be decreased and some seizures allowed— in order to avoid side effects which may be worse than the seizures themselves. In cases that are difficult to control, a great deal of trial and error may be necessary. The patient and the doctor must work together to reach an acceptable medium. Drug therapy may also be supplemented by various diets and/or in some cases surgical treatment.

*   *   *

B. SURGERY

Is Five Centimeters Too Much?

Neil Roberts began having petit mal seizures when he was nine years old. A month later these gave way to psychomotor seizures manifested by momentary states of confusion. Within a year and a half, however, anti-convulsants had brought these seizures under control. Neil suffered no difficulty at all from age eleven to nineteen.

To Neil's shock, during his first year in college his seizures recurred. For a time, increasing his medication brought everything under control. He had no further problem until he was twenty-four. Then seizures began to occur regularly. By the time Neil was twenty-six, he was experiencing about two seizures every week. Unless something drastic was done, he felt that conditions would only continue to worsen.

Because of heavy doses of medication, Neil had more and more difficulty concentrating and reading. Since he was studying psychology, he did a great deal of reading about the brain. He began to question his career stability. He began to doubt his abilities to meet the goals which he had set. It seemed his career would be disrupted by a lifetime of seizures. He realized that he was irritable much of the time and this affected his psychological attitude and outlook. He found that he tended to work at jobs which enabled him to be alone, although he enjoyed other people.

After one and a half years of looking for and failing to find help, Neil found an article about surgery for children with temporal lobe seizures. He began to read more neurological material in the library. He could see his own situation was similar to those described in the literature. He had begun to hyperventilate during the seizures and to have masticatory seizures (chewing and blowing, etc.) The lesions in Neil's brain seemed to influence his psychological state.[102] Was he withdrawing socially? Did he have or would he have a social life that would be worthwhile?

He decided to see a neurosurgeon and find out if an operation was the answer. The neurosurgeon ran twelve tests and found that Neil had a lesion in the anterior temporal lobe of his brain. This could be easily understood because of the type of aura which preceeded his seizures. Neil had a feeling of fear or strangeness prior to a seizure. Because this was the only lesion, and there were no seizures on the other side of the brain, Neil was considered a good candidate for surgery.

It took him several months to come to a firm decision. This was really a major operation. However, Neil finally made up his mind. On November 14th, 1976, he entered the hospital for surgery.

The night before the operation he sat on the side of the bed wondering if he had made the right decision. His girlfriend, Judy, had come with him and talked to the neurologist and the neurosurgeon. What if this operation produced a different person—one she could no longer love? The intern came in with the release form to sign. The fact that the intern had never given such a form to anyone before did not make him feel any better.

Soon it was morning. The nurses were getting him ready for surgery. Someone was sticking him with a needle. Another person was cutting off his hair. Then, he was asleep.

Fifteen minutes later Neil awoke. He was back in his room. When he asked the time, he realized with surprise that five hours had passed. His head hurt. The next day, he sneaked into the bathroom to look at himself in the mirror and saw the brownish stitches on his temple. Fifteen days later he left the hospital.

Neil had planned to meet his mother at the front of the hospital. However, when he was ready to leave, no one was there to wheel him to the door. He took off on his own, a disoriented, disgruntled person. He had felt that the operation would have little or no effect upon him. However, his lack of orientation convinced him that it had not been as simple as he had expected. He wound up at the wrong end of the hospital. After successfully losing himself in the building, he finally arrived at the correct door and went home.

Neil's operation had some disheartening aftereffects.

Two months after the surgery, Neil felt a bone in his cranium move. A bone flap had sunk inwards, leaving an indentation on his forehead which he considers a disfigurement. Seven and a half months after surgery he experienced more complications; minor paralysis of the right forehead and facial muscles, a popping or clicking sensation in the right side of his jaw (probably due to a misalignment of the temporal mandibular joint), and depression. He was not sure how to best deal with these problems. He refused to accept them for a long, long time and sank into depression.

The psychological shock of the surgery took three years to wear off. Now Neil can look back and see that it was worthwhile. He is no longer on medication. His ability to read has improved. He is working full time and going to the university. He received a degree in psychology and is working on a degree in business. With the cessation of seizure activity, life has taken on a new dimension. When I last talked with him in November of 1983, he was considering going to South America.

*   *   *

Surgery is used as treatment for epilepsy only in very selected cases. When the seizures are very disabling because of their frequency and/or severity and cannot be controlled with medication, or when control of seizures can be achieved only by such a dose of medication that it would make the patient incapable of performing his normal intellectual activities, surgery can be considered. Only a few patients have sufficiently localized electrical abnormality to allow the surgeon to remove the part of the brain involved. If the abnormality is generalized, surgical treatment cannot be considered. But, even when there is a well-defined focal abnormality, this must be located in an area of the brain of which the removal will not result in disabling paralysis, speech or memory involvement. Therefore, at the time of this writing, surgery as treatment for seizures is limited to relatively few cases. Several centers are working on new procedures which probably will enlarge the scope of the type of treatment. However, at the moment, these procedures are in an experimental state.[103]

* * *

C. NUTRITION

"Physicians in this century have relearned what physicians of former times have always known: that if any part of the human mechanism is defective, the whole is affected."[104]

In the past few years researchers have been focusing more on nutrition and its interaction for their well-being. Nutrition has become increasingly important to individuals. The food we eat or do not eat can have an important effect on the health of our bodies.

William H. Philpott, M.D., an Oklahoma physician, carries this point further. He suggests that: "Foods, or the lack of them, are closely linked to such degenerative diseases as epilepsy, autism, and cerebral palsy." Philpott contends that problems such as hyperactivity, depression, and inability to control one's emotions and/or behaviour may be traced to certain foods, irritants and chemicals.

Philpott is a member of a field known as "orthomolecular medicine," which deals with metabiology and nutrition. One of the current goals of this field is to replace drugs with other therapies. In other words, good nutritional habits can influence the abilities of the body to compensate for neurological defects. That is where nutritional habits and food come into play.

One of the first things these specialists look for in an impaired or disabled individual is whether reactions are affected by allergic reactions to foods, inhalants or chemicals. They take into consideration the nutritional needs of the individual, as well as his or her need for therapeutic assistance in learning social skills.

In orthomolecular medicine, a great deal of laboratory work is done to give the physician a broader understanding of the makeup of the individual. Special tests for hair particles, blood counts, and bone marrow are among those used.

A specific dietary component under study is B_6 vitamin deficiency, which can be a cause of an abnormal electroencephalogram (EEG) or may lead to epileptic seizures. Allergic reactions to food and chemicals may also induce epileptic seizures.

"Deficiencies of the B complex, especially B_6, and vitamin C produce unhealthy brain functions and predispose patients to maladaptive reactions of the central nervous system. The same is true for minerals. Magnesium, for instance, is one of the most important elements for healthy brain function, and its presence at less than optimal levels can have serious consequences."[105]

In epileptic patients a change in blood sugar can induce a seizure when oxygen is cut off from the brain.[106] Case studies show instances in which a child diagnosed as having psychomotor epilepsy was tested and found to be unable to tolerate various foods. These foods caused the seizures. When the diet was changed, remission of the seizures occurred. The tests which are used in clinics such as the one in Oklahoma test the effects of changes within the environment as reflected in diet, hair and skin.

Allergy-like reactions may excite or inhibit tissues and organs in the body capable of causing seizures. This type of maladaptive reaction has been called the "great masquerader". Depression, hallucination, delusion, perceptual distortions, catatonia, flatness of affect, hyperactivity, etc., are all such reactions.[107]

Proponents of orthomolecular medicine test for patients' reactions to a variety of foods: (1) Foods grown without insecticides; (2) market-grown foods which contain insecticide residues; (3) raw foods; (4) cooked foods; (5) foods with preservatives and colors added. The reaction a person has to these foods can indicate what they may be allergic to.

Allergists are in agreement with physicians who feel that more and better nutritional studies need to be done. These studies will give the physician a broader understanding of the individual and enable him to treat the whole person. Fifty percent of epileptic patients do not require medication when they are put on a diet.[108]

Some neurologists still do not realize the importance allergies can play in epilepsy. If the physician is not able to work out the case by mere food elimination, he may be wise to refer the person to an allergist for further study. In some cases allergies hold the key to treatment.

*　　　*　　　*

D. BIOFEEDBACK

Biofeedback is a relatively new method of self-regulating stress by which the individual monitors and regulates his own biological processes. This may be done by placing mechanisms inside the body (invasive techniques such as electrodes placed within the skin through needles) or using measuring devices applied to the skin (non-invasive techniques such as electrodes which do not break the skin.) Electrical signals are generated by some bodily tissue. These signals are then modified to trigger a visual or auditory display so the individual may have continuous information to control the signal.[109]

Biofeedback is used with many types of disorders including neuromuscular disorders, hyperactivity, hypertension, migraine headaches, cerebral palsy and epilepsy. Certain epileptic patients who have been on biofeedback in the hospital for a time are allowed to go home with a monitoring machine to continue their treatment. In some cases this treatment seems effective for epileptics.[110]

The biofeedback machines are different for various uses of the body. At the present time, they are all fairly expensive. Hopefully, they will go down in price. Some are sold in separate individual units; others, in large units containing 8 or more divisions.

The biolab, which is a machine designed by Barry Sterman, M.D. at the V.A. Hospital in Sepulvada, California is in operation in only a few places in the United States; among them are LaCrosse, Wisconsin and Knoxville, Tennessee. It is capable of measuring at least eight various activities of the body simultaneously through the use of one set of electrodes. Among these are the electroencephalogram, electromylogram, galvonic skin reactor to name a few. Like a computer it works to organize all the material so that the therapist can get a more systematic reading. This biolab machine is set up so that additional monitoring devices may be inserted at a later date to monitor other functions within the body.[111]

Certain brain waves of the epileptic person show an absence of specific 12–14 Hertz (Hz or cycles per second) rhythms and the presence of 4Hz to 7Hz rhythms. This has led researchers to believe that by bringing these specific rhythms to a normal wave length, they might be better able to control seizures. Researchers in biofeedback have focussed on this and sought to convert them both to a normal display.

Three laboratories located in Oklahoma, Tennessee and California deal with the research of sensory motor training (SMR) in epilepsy introduced by the aforementioned B. Sterman, M.D. Research at the laboratories in Tennessee and Oklahoma led to more conclusive methods in treating epilepsy. Joel Lubar, Ph.D. (Tennessee) and William W. Finley, M.D. (Oklahoma)[112] both found that the person with motor involvement in seizures enabled the sensory rhythm training to be more beneficial. Lubar found both excellent and poor results in persons having psychomotor seizures.[113] He feels that akinetic and myoclonic seizures are easiest to treat.

Persons selected for research projects must have been severely debilitated by the concurrence of continuous seizure activity and unsuccessful drug regimens. There must be a reasonable likelihood that they will continue with the therapy. For many severe epileptics, biofeedback offers a hope that the seizure pattern will be resolved or held in check voluntarily. Presently 75% of the people with epilepsy are controled on anti-convulsant therapy. The other 25% are faced with recurring seizures at high rates.[114]

Quy, an English researcher, gives the following three examples of persons treated for biofeedback:

(1) A male, 32 years old with secondary generalized seizures had been treated for twenty-one years. Medication was unsuccessful. The person suffered four tonic-clonic seizures a month. His seizures through biofeedback were reduced by 32%.

(2) A female, 47 years old having a three-year history of primarily generalized epilepsy—tonic-clonic seizures continued. In 1965, she experienced status epilepticus. Her medication was unsuccessful and seizures continued. Presently, the seizures have been relieved by 58% through biofeedback.

(3) A male, 39 years old, suffered from psycho-motor. These were first recorded at age 8. Tonic-clonic in the left side of the body was observed. Psychomotor seizures were preceeded by an aura consisting of a buzzing sound. Reduction rate of seizures was 55%.[115]

Biofeedback is not only used in treatment centers, such as the new ones in Wisconsin and Tennessee, but has also been introduced into some school systems. It is presently used in school systems over the country. Spearfish, South Dakota is one such system. It can be used for activities from biology to artistic expression, even in teaching a prophylactic course in relaxation.[116] The reduction of stress in everyday life has been one of the most beneficial aspects of biofeedback. It is through this, that it is conceivable for persons with epilepsy to benefit the most. Neither the best nor the worst means of treatment, it is used successfully with some patients.

*　　　　*　　　　*

E. THE COMPREHENSIVE EPILEPSY PROGRAM

Station 49

In the United States there are four basic units for comprehensive treatment control of seizures. They are located in Baltimore, Seattle, Los Angeles and Minneapolis. The Comprehensive Treatment Program for adults at the University of Minnesota Hospital-Station 49 is located in Minneapolis, and the program for children is located at Gilette Children's Hospital in Saint Paul. These units were set up primarily for those persons whose recurrent seizures were interfering with their ability to live useful lives. The criteria for selecting a patient for this program is based upon:

1. the degree of difficulty in controlling the seizure
2. difficulty with medication side effects
3. seizures which are difficult to diagnose
4. possibility of surgical treatment

Screening is carefully done by clinicians who are able to discern if the person is a good candidate for the program. People come from all over the United States to participate in this program. Since its inception in November, 1976 more than 400 patients have been treated and discharged from this unit. The approximate stay is six weeks. On admission, these patients averaged nine seizures per week. Two years after discharge 50% reported that their seizure control was much improved, and 25% reported that they were seizure free. 25% reported no significant change. Overall, seizure frequency was 1.3 per week. Most subjects reported substantial improvements in employment and independent living.[117]

The program at the University of Minnesota is quite unique in its approach. In addition to highly specialized medical and surgical care, the psychosocial and vocational needs of the patient are also treated. A team of neurologists, nurses, social workers, psychologists and other specialists respond to the problems of each patient.[118]

Through proper diagnosis, treatment and evaluation it is possible to treat the person in the wisest and best manner. Vital data provided from video-EEG and clinical observations enable the team to properly identify the individual type of seizure and provide the best anticonvulsants available. The aim of the medication treatment program is to provide the optimal seizure control with a minimum of medication. Professional opinions regarding the feasibility of surgery are based partially on this data.

The impact of the disorder upon the social and vocational outlook of the individual cannot be overlooked. Psychological, social and vocational evaluation includes individual and family counseling. Group therapy is provided. Patient education classes about epilepsy are conducted five days per week to increase the social awareness and understanding of the individual. Vocational planning is guided by careful work evaluation. These programs enable the individual to build a better lifestyle for themselves. When the team feels that the individual is ready to resume his/her role in the community, it shares its results and makes specific recommendations to the individual and their family. Written reports are sent to the primary physician and referring agency. The patient is asked to return for one clinic visit after discharge. Care is then referred back to the physician of the patient's choice. Continuing neurological care is available at the patient's request.[119]

Before coming to this program, most people have gone to many other programs which failed to help. Visiting with two patients at Station 49, I got the impression that this program was different from any that they had previously participated in. They seemed relieved that their condition was finally being treated as a disorder rather than a disease. The 50/50 ratio of men and women helped maintain an equal balance which provided a better social relationship and a more realistic situation. This in turn prepared the people to relate better to real life situations which they would be facing upon their dismissal from the program. As Larry commented, "When there are men and women, there are less arguments among the individuals."

Although both Tom and Larry have had epilepsy for approximately twenty-five years, they were different ages at the onset of epilepsy. Fortunately both have supportive families. Tom has had the disorder since birth. Larry's condition began at age seventeen. This has made a difference in the manner that they accepted the disorder. Tom has lived with the problem all of his life and has adapted to it out of necessity. The fact that it struck Larry in his late teen's has made it a problem to accept. This is the age when young people are first learning to drive and seeking work. Jobs are difficult for persons with epilepsy to find.

Tom was a participant in the program five years ago. At

that time physicians were trying to control his seizures through medication. He has been in Minneapolis three weeks at the time of this writing. He is back anticipating surgery as a possible means of control. Since he has been here, his medication has been drastically cut. This has enabled the physicians to observe his seizures. (Unfortunately most neurologists seldom see their patient having the seizure. Station 49 is set up so that individuals may be monitored and observed during seizures and tested in numerous ways. This provides a better foundation for treatment. Most persons do not know what occurs during their seizures.) Tom is presently undergoing several kinds of tests and carefully recording the seizures which do occur. He was on 1600 mg. of Tegretol and 700 mg. of Dilantin when he entered the program. It should be emphasized that the practice of reducing medication in order to witness seizures should occur only in very specialized and prepared centers, such as Station 49.

Tom has psychomotor seizures, during which he usually becomes "super strong." On occasion he has kicked his mother. This violence that occurs during the seizures bothers him because he is a gentle person. Characteristics of his seizure include body jerks, right tremor and loss of balance. He always loses consciousness. This is one reason that the requirement of wearing safety helmets while participating in this program is very important. During the time when the physicians are changing the medications, it is quite likely that the person may fall during the seizure. The helmet shields the person from harming themselves should they fall. Even though the helmets are worn, some individuals who fall a great deal have still hurt themselves.

Every individual reacts to drugs differently. Tom has found that Mysoline causes him to feel suicidal. Sodium valproate causes him to lose his appetite and complain of a sore throat.

Tom feels that his treatment at Station 49 has helped him to associate with other people and to explain what it is like to have epilepsy. He has learned how to act and react with people, how to explain his problem to them, and how to be more assertive. Group communicators help patients to understand their problems and to learn to deal with them. Independent living skills are taught in an easy relaxed manner. Tom is no longer forced to stay in a bed with side-rails drawn up during his stint in this hospital. On Friday nights each person is supposed to fix his own supper. Everyone is required to do his own laundry. Everyone here has the same problem, only in varying degrees. No one feels "different".

They have become more relaxed and developed more friendships. Both Larry and Tom feel that developing new friends is important. Larry emphasized the point that "before coming here, he felt that he was the only person with epilepsy." Since the disorder started in his late teens it was difficult to accept. His family was supportive, yet some of his in-laws thought for a long time that he was making things up. It wasn't until he fell and hurt himself on a gravel drive that they took him seriously.

"I was considered the fall down drunk," Larry said. Of course, this has had a devastating effect on his self-esteem. Since being at Station 49, he has been able to see a lot of other types/styles of seizures. This has broadened his acceptance of himself and given him support which has enabled him to accept the problem. Before, he had denied the problem. Now he is much more open toward the situation he finds himself in. "I appreciate this place. Other places that I have been in have confined me to a bed as if I were ill. Here you are on your own. You have to get up and dress in the morning. There are other people to visit with and observe. There is therapy that enables you to better understand yourself, and your ability to deal with reality. Before coming here, I felt sorry for myself. I *KNEW* that I was the *ONLY PERSON WITH EPILEPSY* in the world. Of course, I'm not. Until I came here and saw other people having more problems than I, I really felt sorry for myself. In fact, I tried to deny that there really was a problem. None of the doctors I saw seemed to be able to help. Nothing seemed to work out. Jobs when they did occur put me with the public. I was never certain when my seizures would strike. Consequently, I lived in fear of recrimination. This put me under unneeded stress which only made matters worse. Station 49 has changed this. In only one and a half weeks I have learned to accept myself. It's like being a bachelor again. You have to depend upon yourself.

"They have changed the medication now after only a short time. They are finding small blood vessels at the top of my skull which was unusual. At other hospitals they were unable to do this. Next week, I should receive the results of my tests and for the first time I will know what type of seizures I actually do have. For the first time I am really optimistic about life!"

*　　　　*　　　　*

F. GENETIC ASPECTS

Research

A thoughtful review of the genetic process and its underlying philosophy has been presented by two leading researchers, Julius and Katherine Metrakos. They have demonstrated the following two things in their studies: (1) The rate of epilepsy in the next-of-kin of children admitted with convulsions to Montral Pediatric Hospital is higher than the next-of-kin of other children. (2) A study of EEGs of the next-of-kin of epileptic patients suggests that generalized epilepsy is inherited by a dominant gene of low penetrance.[120] This means that even though many people do not have epileptic symptoms they carry the abnormal dominant gene, and may pass the gene and the disorder on to some of their children. Other scientists feel that epilepsy more often involves the influence of a multi-complex of genes, rather than a single gene of inheritence. Dr. Metrakos suggests that:

> However, when it is recalled that no gene acts solely by itself but is dependent upon the whole genotype of probably some 10,000 gene pairs, it is unnecessary to mention that biochemical products of each gene interact, directly or indirectly with the biochemical products of all other genes of the individual. Modern gene concepts state that all major action is delicately balanced by a number of controlling genes. Thus although a single major gene may be responsible for the contrencephalic EEG trait a number of other genes may be controlling such factors as its variability in age of onset, sex distribution, and severity into typical and atypical.

Why is the disease so common? What is the relative fertility of affected and unaffected individuals? Do genetic carriers show hybrid vigor? Are there any racial or ethnic differences? At the moment there are no clear answers to many of these questions.

The present approach of epilepsy has been described as the *brute force approach* (surgery) and the *trial and error approach* (anti-convulsant therapy). These two approaches will undoubtedly continue to serve the epileptic well for many years to come. However, if certain forms of epilepsy can be traced to genes, then an understanding of their biosynaptic pathways becomes essential for a more scientific program of therapy. Just as genetic blocks (absent enzymes) identified in phenylketonuria (PKU) and galactosemia, so too, in genetic epilepsy, it may be possible some day to identify some forms of genetic deficiencies.

Investigations conducted in the last 15 years have added substantially to the conclusion that hereditary facts are implicated in the etiology of epilepsy. The result of studies of many investigators have compounded this evidence. Thus the problem is no longer whether or not genes are important in the epilepsies, but rather (1) to identify which genes are actually in which of the epilepsies and, (2) to determine which of these genes may be common to more than one type of epilepsy.[121]

Reasonably good data show that brothers and sisters of probands (persons who first have the disorder in the family) run a higher risk of contracting epilepsy or epileptic traits than do other children.[122] It has been learned that persons who are epileptic and whose family may have had carriers of epilepsy are more difficult to treat. They suffer from leukopenia (low white blood corpuscles) and react adversely to many anti-convulsants which the normal person has no difficulty using.[123]

Genetic researchers are learning more about the important part genes play in the make-up of the brain.[124] It may well be biochemists who unlock the genetic components of epilepsy. A simple explanation is unlikely due to the vast differences between individual epileptics. Evidence suggests that there is not one gene which will act to control all epilepsies, but that there are several.[125] Studies conducted by Lennox on 20,000 relatives of 4,231 epileptic patients show a prevalence of epilepsy in near relatives of the essential or idiopathic group of 3.6% as compared to 1.8% of the near relatives of the symptomatic or acquired group. These findings indicate the genetic factor was more important in idiopathic as compared to symptomatic groups.[126]

In a collaborative study with Janz,[127] C. K. Benninger et. al., studied the influence of parental types of epilepsy on the frequency of spike-wave discharges in EEGs. In children of parents with contrencephalic types of seizures (absence petit mal, massive bilateral myoclonus, with or without grand mal) they found generalized spike wave in the EEG twice as often compared with children of parents with focal seizures (with or without grand mal). Moreover, there were more often SW discharges (20%) compared with offspring of parents with sleep grand mal (13%).[128]

For many years, the question of genetics and its relationship to epilepsy has been a subject of interest and controversy. Swedish laws promulgated in 1757 and remaining in effect until the twentieth century forbade marriage by epileptic patients.[129] German authorities during the Nazi regime attempted to sterilize epileptics.[130] Similar laws regarding sterilization remained in effect in fourteen American states as late as 1968.[131] Until quite recently, there was no proof of any genetic tie, although the scientists did consider that epilepsy had a genetic component. Specialists haven't really decided whether epilepsy is genetically passed on. It is safe to say that if both parents have epilepsy the risk that the children will have epilepsy is doubled. The type of spike on an EEG can be a determining factor in devining genetic aspects.[132]

Our bodies are composed of genetic components known as genotypes and phenotypes. The genotype refers to the genetic makeup of an individual. Its potential for development may differ with varying environmental circumstances.[133] In contrast, the phenotype is the visible physical manifestation of the combination of genes and environment. Character traits result from the interaction of genotypes and the environment. A person with a given genotype may have a different phenotype. He will be a different person if placed in a different environment. The phenotype is distinguished by visible characteristics, not by hereditary or genetic traits.

The person in the family who is the first to contract or display epilepsy is spoken of as the "proband." It is he or she who introduces the disorder to the family. Researcher V. Elving Anderson of the University of Minnesota has the following points to offer:

"Genetic counseling is a useful and important means of appraising familial links in epilepsy, and should be part and parcel of every patient's management.

"The goal of genetic counseling is to provide individuals

and families with the information and understanding they need in order to make informed choices about future reproduction. In order to diagnose properly the possibility of genetic occurrence, the following should be gathered in clinical sessions:

> A 'pedigree' chart listing the patient and all immediate relatives (parents, children, siblings);
> Notation of other relatives who have epilepsy or an associated disorder;
> Information on any intermarriage of relatives, in which an autosomal recessive disorder is possible in the offspring.

"If the situation is mild, we usually think that we are dealing with a problem which involves many genes. If it is severe, it is more likely that there is a single major chromosome anomaly, birth trauma or other such factor.[134]

"By age fifteen, about one percent of the population will have developed recurrent seizures. By age forty, the diagnosis is about two percent: by age seventy, about 3.5 percent.[135] For further information regarding genetic traits see '100 Mendelian traits—Table 1'."

Genetic Counseling and the Role of the Counselor

There are two groups of people who come for assistance to the genetic counselor: those who seek counseling after the epilepsy has already occurred in their children, and those who seek counseling because of knowledge that there is some serious problem or genetic disorder in their family history.

The genetic counselor explains to the family what the disorder is, what risks it entails, and what possibilities exist to resolve these risks. A couple who has seizure disorders yet desires a family may seek counseling to obtain information regarding the amount of risk involved, as well as the possibility of resolution of the problems they may face in the future. Counselors are aware of the social stigma attached to epilepsy, and are able to help the prospective parents consider all the effects before reaching a decision. In some ways counselors are similar to social workers; they are able to explain the disorder in rational terms which do not overwhelm the prospective parents. They may encourage them to return for future assistance if needed because some parents have a great difficulty accepting and coping with the reality of epilepsy within their own family.[136]

Any genetic counselor who merely gives facts lacks both compassion and the foresight necessary to help the parents through the five stages of grief. The parent may first deny that any problem exists; this may be followed by depression upon the realization that epilepsy does pose a problem to their child. Anger at the situation, followed by rejection of the child are normal reactions. It is up to the counselor to help the parent turn this negative feeling into one of acceptance of the child and the situation.[137]

Epilepsy acts as a pebble dropped into a pool. It sheds out ripples to other people. When the winds of doubt and denial blow harshly, the ripples are no longer calm circles. Genetic counselors must work with the entire family. The disorder's effects may be felt not only by the person with the disorder, but also family, friends, colleagues and neighbors.

Acceptance by those who do work and live with epileptics is an essential system of support. It helps the epileptic person work out his/her own problems. Without such a system, they may feel incapable and lose the self-esteem so vital to leading a productive life.

Genetic counseling is available to most people in clinics throughout the country. For women in their childbearing years whose families have a history of epilepsy, counseling may help them realize that anti-convulsant therapy may be detrimental to the fetus. Mothers who might otherwise breast-feed their babies are generally advised not to do so. If the child is breast fed, they run the risk of being given a high amount of anti-convulsants through the milk, thereby making them drowsy and irritable.

Genetic counseling may act as a stabilizing factor to enable persons to deal with situations in rational manner. As research continues to unravel the mysteries of epilepsy, more and more will be learned about just what part heredity does play in epilepsy. Genetic counseling makes it possible for people to accept their epilepsy, rather than hide the fact that they do have the disorder. In the past, when the fact has been hidden, the problem has turned up in succeeding generations without any knowledge that it had occurred in preceding generations.

*   *   *

III

A Parent's Viewpoint

Parents live with their children twenty-four hours a day; they know their idiosyncrasies better than anyone else. Although they may have difficulty accepting the fact that their child has epilepsy, they might learn to cope with the situation. What follows are the personal experiences of several such parents.

A. P.M.

About eight years ago when Nancy was three years old, I discovered her staring straight ahead, unaware of what was going on around her. I took her to the doctor, who told me that these spells were petit mal seizures. The word "seizures" gave me chills. She went to the doctor so often for blood tests and EEGs that I wondered if they would ever find the right amount of medication to control her seizures.

I felt all torn up inside every time that I saw Nancy go into a seizure. When they finally did get them controlled I was so happy! It seemed to me that petit mal seizures were not as bad as other kinds of seizures, but I still felt that seizures of any kind were a very bad thing.

In March of 1977, I got a call from the school telling me that Nancy had had a grand mal seizure. I did not want to believe it. I was hoping so much that she would outgrow her seizures. I took her to the doctor who put her on another kind of medication, but three months later Nancy had another grand mal seizure. Nancy was playing outside. I looked to see if she was playing nicely and behaving herself, as most mothers do. She was having a great time and seemed O.K. Just a few minutes later, my neighbor came knocking at my door to say that something was wrong with Nancy. The minute I went to the door, I knew what was wrong. It was the first time that I had ever seen Nancy, or anyone, having a grand mal seizure. She looked like a wet dishrag lying in the yard. I cannot even describe how I felt when I saw her that way. From this experience I learned that seizures can happen any time, and very quickly.

Anyone who has not known my daughter would never know that she is an epileptic because, as I said before, her seizures are controlled with the medication that she takes.

It just does not seem fair to those who have epilepsy. To me, it is as if something has been taken away from them that does not deserve to be taken away.

*   *   *

B. PILOT PARENTS

Lisa's brain was damaged at birth. When her head was crowning, the nurses pushed her back in and held her there fifteen minutes until the doctor arrived. A lack of oxygen resulted. Seizures began immediately. Her legs would grow rigid and jerk for a few seconds. Her eyes would roll backwards into her head.

Epilepsy has meant many sleepless nights for us. For the first three months after she began to take phenobarbital, our daughter was awake day and night.

One of our biggest problems has been competent babysitters. Some neighbors (adults and children) have teased Lisa, though most people have accepted her. Nursery school teachers have been very cooperative. She will be tested in a preschool assessment program this fall, finish this year in nursery school, and start public school next fall. I am anticipating a good year.

Lisa seems to be developing quite normally. She does have difficulty with her ears. At the moment she has tubes in them so that they will drain properly. Aside from this, she is a normal little girl. She has likes and dislikes just like anyone else; she would love to have a canopy bed; she does not like to be spanked. Periodically she has nightmares about the devil. Her classmates now understand what may happen and can treat her like any other school child.

At first, my husband withdrew from Lisa. He would not communicate with her, play with her or assist me in my decisions involving her. When they were in public together he would make her "perform" or show off how much she could do. Since our involvement in Pilot Parents, he has improved tremendously. Now they work and play together well. Pilot Parents is a support group for parents of handicapped children here in Duluth. Parents undergo training on how to communicate effectively with doctors and other professionals. They share common experiences and are made aware of resources available in the community. This group has led us to be more accepting of our child's problems.

Involvement in the local epilepsy league also helped me to learn more about the disorder and resources available. Volunteering my services made me feel that I was at least doing something for Lisa. Contact with other parents and their children and seeing how they interact with each other has also been very helpful.

I would like to see more public education about epilepsy. I see the main problem as employment and general acceptance of persons with epilepsy. This is something that we will have to face. Although we realize that there will be things which Lisa may not be able to do, we are thankful that her seizures are as controlled as they are.

* * *

C. SUNRISE CONTROVERSY

Jean Anne is a pleasant nine-year-old brown-eyed, black-haired fourth grader. She enjoys her school work. She has completed one year in the Title I program and is presently getting special education through the program at the school. At the end of the 1976 school term her teachers felt that she might have petit mal epilepsy. She had a tendency to stare blankly into space at intermittent intervals. She did not seem aware of what had been said. Although tests seemed inconclusive, Jean Anne was placed on phenobarbital three times a day for eighteen months. She was taken off medication in December of 1977. She has had no major seizures since that time. All traces of epilepsy have vanished. Her work has improved. Jean Anne no longer stares blankly.

"We have always taken a wait and see outlook," her father said. "I felt that she had had a learning problem when the testing was begun. She reads quite well. She likes multiplication, but could not add and subtract, just multiply."

Jean Anne has two older siblings, fifteen and twelve. They have learned a great deal since their sister has had epilepsy. The entire family has. From the beginning, these parents were helped to understand the disorder through their contacts with the local Epilepsy League. It was apparent that there was a good relationship in the family. At one time they tried to form a parents group which would meet and discuss seizure problems.

When asked if they had discussed Jean Anne's problems with others, they indicated that relatives did not really want to discuss the possibility of epilepsy. People skirted the issue gingerly. At school, only a few teachers were told of the situation. Jean Anne's mother commented that at first she had wondered. "Why did this happen to us?" That question sounds familiar. Parents of children with problems usually wonder this at some point. She confessed this kind of reaction to the news of her daughter's problem, that she "kind of went to pieces." However, she eventually realized that the actual problem was not nearly as unsolvable as it had first seemed. "It was a relief to know what the problem was, so that we could deal with it," she said emphatically.

Jean Anne enjoys sports and other activities most children do. She is a very active child. She told me how she had been fingerprinted earlier this week so that she could be in the junior police. She was quite proud of her badge, which she wore on her skirt.

She seemed to understand her condition; she told me she would be glad to come over and discuss it again if I liked. This young girl has not had any really severe seizures. She accepts what comes, and it has ceased to be a problem. She is now free of any medication and her seizures are completely under control. Although it does not happen often, children can grow out of petit mal epilepsy.

*   *   *

D. STATUS EPILEPTICUS IN SISTERS

Two of our three daughters have status epilepticus. We found it very difficult to accept. They also have other disabling conditions. I accepted my daughter's visual limitations, her physical disability and retardation; but seizures were an unknown quantity which I could not accept or prepare for. I could not control them or make them go away. Not knowing what caused them was also disturbing. None of our family has any known history of epilepsy. The visual limitation was caused by a recessive gene. The girls, aged ten and eleven, did not acquire the seizures until seventeen months and two years old respectively. Alicia's problem was externally caused; DeAnne's interally caused due to the lack of development of her brain. Yet both had the same type of seizure pattern.

Our children's epilepsy is different from most. Status epilepticus is a very serious type of epilepsy. It can result in death if the proper procedures are not followed. It may be provoked by a brain injury or poisoning; or by the withdrawal of a drug.

Alicia lost her eyesight through an unsuccessful corneal transplant. Evidently, there is some scar tissue or lesion in the brain's visual area that could be a partial source of her seizures. She is visually disabled and considered functionally retarded. Her seizures began when she was eighteen months old. All of her visual signs disappeared during the corneal transplant. The doctors did not expect her to live through the night. Three weeks later, her temperature dropped and her entire body reacted to whatever caused the seizure, which was the first of many.

Periodically, she did have seizures. After the operation, she was started on phenobarbital. This caused hyperactivity. It took some time to arrive at a medication which would hold the seizures in check. Dilantin did not work very well either. So we tried Meberal, which seems to be more effective. It will soon be three years since her last seizure. During the time they were most frequent, they occurred about once a week. Just before she has her seizures, Alicia complains of headaches in the top of her head. This serves as a warning for the intense seizure which follows and gives me an opportunity to prepare for the seizure.

DeAnne had brain damage. When the physician found that her brain was not completely formed, he gave her extensive tests. Intellectually she is fine, but she does not get messages to the right limbs. Consequently, she has difficulty using her right arm and trouble walking. She also suffers from status epilepticus. Her seizures are never the same. They can be Jacksonian or grand mal, or a combination. In each seizure her eyes switch to one side before she goes into a comatose state. She does not come out of it until she is given Valium intravenously or intramuscularly. I give it intramuscularly. This comatose state can be most dangerous. DeAnne's seizures do not happen frequently. The most frequent was six a year. Regulation of medication played an important part in decreasing these. She is on 200 mg. of Dilantin per day. The last seizure was a couple of months ago. She was totally in control. She was able to communicate that she was about to have a seizure. She remained conscious, although she had trouble breathing. I gave her 10mg of Valium before taking her to the hospital emergency ward.

Our older daughter Kathryn had only one seizure. She is now thirteen. This occurred after a pneumoencephalogram. My first reaction was shock, fear, helplessness. What had happened? I thought that she was dying. They put her on phenobarbital and then discontinued the drug when she was five years old. A fever had caused the seizures.

It has taken me eleven years to acquire the philosophy I now have. No one has a crystal ball which will tell the future. I am thankful for every day in which our children do not have seizures. If they have one, it is a part of their life so I have to accept it and go on from there. I was a "basket-case" for a long time. Once I drove to the hospital holding one child and driving on the freeway while the other had a seizure during the entire trip. At the time, I could only think of getting help. It was not rational behavior.

I used to call the school repeatedly to tell them how to reach me in case the children had a seizure. I felt as restricted as if I were on parole. I finally decided that the school personnel were getting tired of my calling, so I called the doctor and convinced him to write them giving permission to take the children to the hospital and to give medication when necessary. This letter lifted a burden from me.

The experiences which we have had with our children's teachers have been mostly positive. One teacher wanted to have DeAnne use her bad hand, however, I told her that it would do no good to strengthen it. It must be treated as a helper. Let her use the one which worked best for her. The teachers who work with our children have found them a challenge and have met this challenge admirably.

I try not to keep my children from participating in most things. I have a hang-up about taking the younger children to Valley Fair, a nearby amusement park. However, other people do too. I insist that they go places with someone else. I feel better if the children are not alone. The eleven year old (DeAnne) is able to handle herself. They are all able to make responsible decisions.

Parents should not be overprotective. They should treat their children as normally as possible, being as least restrictive as possible. Children should be looked at first as individuals, then as people with problems.

There are no easy answers about treatment for epilepsy. My husband and I did not agree on the medical treatment. At one time, my husband was extremely negative about doctors. I was between the doctor and my husband. I don't know how much this had to do with our marriage falling apart. At the present time, we are in the midst of a divorce.

I believe that it is fair to say that once the correct medication has been instituted, the children's seizures will be fairly well controlled. The possibility of a seizure is something that I must live with and I am gradually growing more able to do so. I must confess that I do not want to think about puberty. Perhaps the seizures will only reoccur. It frightens me.

I hope that other parents are better informed about the general nature of epilepsy than we were. It is the lack of knowledge which breeds fear and insecurity. Lack of knowledge makes it difficult to accept the nature of the children's seizures.

*　　　　*　　　　*

E. TIM'S HELMET

Our son is almost twenty years old and his seizures have not been controlled for the past eight years. Tim is the youngest child in the family; both older daughters are married and have their own families. He is very close to us. Since he has no friends his own age, he spends all of his leisure time at home. I sometimes feel that we should be freer as a couple now that he is grown; yet, I feel guilty about leaving him alone. Friends ask us out; their children are busy going here and there. When I go, I keep thinking about our son home alone.

On the other hand, Tim never expects us to stay home

with him. He encourages us to go out. He is very independent although he has lost the friends who were his age. Tim seems to lean toward older, more understanding adults. He wears a helmet at all times for protection. He really feels that people his age are making fun of him. Many actually do make wisecracks as they walk or ride by.

Adult neighbors seem very concerned and understanding but I do not think his teachers were in school. Tim did have counselors who helped him adjust. I understand now at the Junior High level they have an Adaptive Physical Education Class. I wish that they had had it when he was that age.

I often wondered what life would be like when Tim graduated from high school a year ago. At the present time, through Vocational Rehabilitation, he is working four hours a day with the Douglas County Citizens for the Retarded as an assistant coach for the Special Olympics. He started taking two courses at college this fall through Vocational Rehabilitation. He is a changed person. He takes pride in having a job and seems to look forward to each day.

I guess the only thing that I can say is that the public should know more about the problem—especially young adults. In our case, many young people make fun of his helmet. I am sure that they do not realize why he wears it.

I would suggest that parents try not to smother their children. Our child could never use the excuse for not attending church, school, etc. He was expected by both his father and myself to get up in the morning and go to school even though many times we were called to the school because of a seizure. Many times he even fell and cut his head open before he started wearing the helmet. Even then, he returned the next day as usual. Never give up. Never give up! Always have hope that seizures will be controlled.

I certainly do feel upset at times over the problems which Tim has had to face. On the other hand, I try to tell myself that things could be worse. He still has the ability to feed and clothe himself. Time is on his side; science continues to find new drugs.

*　　　*　　　*

IV

Epilepsy in the Schools

In talking with teachers, I've met few who have had a great deal of exposure to children with seizures in their classes. Although children with epilepsy are in the classroom, different school districts seem to react to the situation in different ways, some facing the problems more responsibly than others.

In one school district in northern Minnesota, the school nurse issues a first-aid box to each teacher at the beginning of the year. The first-aid box contains explicit instructions for handling seizures. This school has been quite active in promoting an understanding of seizure and other neurological disorders.

School is one of the first places where children come in contact with people outside their family circle. It is important that they feel accepted and liked in these formative years. How the teacher prepares the class for any seizure a child may have makes a great deal of difference. The stigma which is all too often associated with epilepsy can only be erased through better education programs, even for the youngest among us.

A. STORIES FROM TEACHERS

I

Mrs. S.: I had two children in my classroom who had epilepsy. I teach the second grade. The first thing that I did was to contact the Minnesota Epilepsy League and have them send out a film that children would understand. Although it lasted only five minutes, it gave a good description of what should be done if the child had a seizure. We talked about epilepsy in the classroom and tried to prepare the children for the seizures if and when they came. However, the child did not have one. We also had a lot of input from the children in describing seizures they saw, perhaps in a grocery store or other place of business. This was a good learning experience for them.

In the second instance, I also prepared the children by telling them about seizures and the proper assistance to give if they occurred. The child that we had was only there a few months. She was in a foster home, because her parents could not deal with her seizures. The only seizure she had was on a day when I was at home sick with the flu. My substitute was not prepared, but carried on fairly well. She called the school nurse and they needed to take the child to the hospital for some reason. It was a serious seizure. Although the children were a little less secure in my absence, they carried on quite well.

I believe that these children need a lot of love and my policy is to be very open with the children. I try to listen to the parents and get as much input as possible from them. They generally know the newest techniques. I stress with my children the importance of understanding these children and seeing them for the people that they are. I don't want my children to taunt them unthinkingly and I try to prevent this by teaching the children that this is the thing which will hurt the children with epilepsy the most. I stress the importance of their friendship and understanding. Although the second-graders are young, they can do helpful things if they are taught to understand the epileptic rather than gawk at them.

*   *   *

II

Judy H.: Working with kindergarteners as I do, you might say that the children I deal with are immature. Kindergarten level parents have closed their eyes to the problems and in some cases don't accept it. So far, we have had one child who had epilepsy. I was the one who recognized the problem and suggested that the parent see a neurologist. By recognizing the child's staring spells for what they were, we were able to get assistance at an early age. This is one reason why it's so important for teachers to be aware of the warning signals of epilepsy.

*   *   *

III

Mrs. V.: Until you have actually been in the situation of having the child have seizures during your class, you don't know exactly how you will react. Most assuredly, it's important to remain calm and know that you must let the seizure run its course. In most instances, there is no need to contact a doctor for a minor seizure.

*   *   *

IV

Betty: I work in a school which deals specifically with children who have a low I.Q. However, even there I was amazed at the class' response when Martha had her first seizure. One boy, who ordinarily has never been helpful, stopped his work and came over to help me. When she had her first seizure, I was terrified. It took a bit before I remembered that I must stay calm. Most of the children paid no attention to the seizure. This would not be true in a regular class; however, I cannot stress enough proper understanding and acceptance on the part of the teacher. By the end of the year, I thought nothing of her seizures, since she had them quite frequently.

*   *   *

V

Mary Jo: In the program that I am involved in, dealing mainly with young adults who are referred to us directly through the courts, the regular mainstream teacher is not always aware that there is a problem. Only when the person feels that they can trust their teacher, are they likely to relay the information that they have epilepsy. I cannot stress the importance of knowing that there is a problem. Our biggest problem with the student is not knowing when they are experiencing complex partial seizures and when they have been smoking pot. Smoking pot also seems to have an effect on their medication. We have never been certain what has caused certain unusual behaviors. Otherwise the student was treated the same as other students. One thing that I will say is that we have been told via the back route. The school nurse and mainstream teachers do not know of the situation. It's really too bad that there isn't a little more openness on the subject.

Experiences in school affect a child's life for a long time to come. In order to make school a positive experience for the epileptic child, it is very important that teachers understand and accept epilepsy for what it really is.

Grand mal seizures during which the person falls to the floor in a convulsive state may frighten the other children at school unless they have been prepared for the possibility of this happening. Psychomotor seizures are less recognizable and may be viewed by the teacher as insolence or inappropriate behavior on the part of the student. Petit mal seizures in which the child stares or appears to be daydreaming last only a few seconds and may be completely missed unless one is looking for their occurrence. In Holdworth and Whitman's 1974 study, 42 percent of epileptic children attending ordinary schools were described as markedly inattentive.[138] A child may be reprimanded time and again for staring into space and failing to answer a question during one of these momentary lapses.

The manner in which a seizure is handled should be consistent between home and school. It is important for the teacher and parents to jointly set up a program for the child which will be effective if a seizure occurs during school. This cannot be accomplished unless parents share what they know about the seizure pattern of their child with teachers. To be more effective, a teacher must be aware of the warning signals which may precede a seizure, as well as what should be done during the actual seizure. If the teacher records the seizures which do occur, the physician may be better able to measure the effectiveness of the medication used in therapy.

School nurses, teachers and administrators should become familiar with the drugs most often administered to children—Phenobarbital, Dilantin and Zorantin—as well as the side effects which generally accompany these drugs. They include drowsiness, lethargy, hyperactivity, loss of muscular coordination, double vision, convulsion, slurred speech, nausea, increase in body hair, tremor, anemias, sleep disturbance, loss of appetite, stomach aches and gum swelling. The adjustment to drug levels in children is an ongoing process, and school personnel must be alert to possible side effects. Any side effect noted should be reported to the parents.[139] Their presence may suggest another look at medication schedules is apropos.

*   *   *

B. LEGISLATION AND THE SCHOOLS

Among those questions parents consistently ask educators and therapists is "How can we assure our child equal education under the law?"

Legislation has been written to provide for equal education of all children in the "least restrictive alternative" for the good of the child. (Subpart D of Sec. 504 of the Voc. Rehab. Act of 1973 and in the Sec. 124A4 of PL 94-142.) However for the legislation to bring about the desired goal: equal education under the law, proper implementation must be achieved.

In order to insure equal education, the history behind the law must be kept in perspective. Those persons responsible for implementation are: teachers, psychologists, administrators, therapists and parents, all members of the implementing community. [140]

To some, the new law has been misconstrued to mean that all handicapped children, regardless of the severity of the handicap, are to be placed in regular classroom programs. To others, the law means that all handicapped children are to be placed in self-contained special education classes. Both are extreme. What the law calls for is a broadening role of the "school community in providing the best possible program for the individual child in the most advantageous setting." This is called mainstreaming. One effect of the Act is to bring a closer alignment between parents and teachers as they ponder the best way to meet the law, a goal that is desirable for all. [141] It is possible to arrive at the best program for the individual child only if parents, teachers and therapists work together in a unified effort. Without their cooperation this law cannot be effective. Parents need to participate fully in the writing of the Individual Education Play (IEP) in order to provide the teacher with necessary information. As much knowledge about the child as possible should be incorporated into the plan. Consequently, the input from physicians, therapists, parents and teachers should be looked upon as an asset needed to provide the best program for the child. Teachers will be able to do a better job if they know and understand the child's actions and interactions and the characteristics of the neurological disorder from which the child suffers, as well as their own reactions to situations.

A specific definition of the Individual Education Plan (IEP) is included with the Act (PL 94-142, 1975, Sec 4.2.19).

> A written statement for each handicapped child developed in any meeting by a representative of the local educational agency or an immediate educational unit who shall be qualified to provide, or supervise the provision of, specifically designed instruction to meet the unique needs of the handicapped child, the teachers, the parents or guardians of such children, and whenever appropriate, such child, which statement shall include (A) a statement of the present levels of educational performance of each child, (B) a statement of annual goals, including short term instructional objectives; (C) a statement of the specific educational services to be provided to each child, and the extent to which such children will be able to participate in regular educational programs, (D) projected data for initiation and anticipated duration of such services, and appropriate objective criteria and evaluation procedures and

schedules for determining, on at least an annual basis, whether instructional objectives are being achieved.[142]

The IEP is used to set up the best program for the child. The teachers/psychologists should write an Individual Educational Program which they feel provides the best educational goals for the child. The parents must approve of it. If they do not, it must be changed so that they are satisfied. Parents have the right to talk with the school board and school examiners if they are not satisfied with the hearing proceedings of the IEP or the final written conclusion of this document. The most effective way, as far as challenging the school, may be to find a common pattern among a large population that is affected and enact a class action suit.

Courses of action available to parents

Independent evaluation

Under the Act, school systems must pay for testing. If a hearing examiner requests an evaluation, the school system must pay for testing. If parents request a second examination, they must pay for it.

Hearing

Independent evaluation will always be used as part of the hearing examiner's decision. The hearing examiner is the person who makes sure that the child is adequately tested.

You must *receive notice* of the hearing. You have 45 days before the statute of limitations runs out. You are free to bring counsel and cross examine the witnesses. If you do nothing, there will be no need to request a hearing and the material will automatically pass into law.

Administrative appeal

This is the last step prior to filing a complaint with the office of civil rights. If this is to be used, you should start at the local level, then the state board of education. All avenues of appeal and/or negotiation must be exhausted before you go to a court hearing to file a complaint.

Complaint

To Federal offices of *civil rights*.

Lawsuits

P.L. 94-194 laid out the ground rules for education of all children. The real push for this law began with the Vocational Rehabilitation Act of 1973, Sec 503/504. This law provides that society must provide handicapped persons with appropriate education. It was especially important since the implementation of Public Law 94-142. Sec. 504 threatened to cut off Federal financial assistance if these conditions were not met. Through this action children who needed special aid were mainstreamed into regular classes. In many cases, the teachers were not ready or prepared for mainstreaming when it first began. With the enactment of Public Law 94-142 they needed a better understanding of the problem children faced, and they needed this understanding immediately. The entirely new outlook on education which suddenly became necessary stunned many classroom teachers.

Minnesota state legislation has set up a model that divides students into six different categories or levels as listed below. Other states may have a different way of dividing the children into levels, but the effect is the same. Most children with epilepsy are able to go into the regular classroom without significant difficulties. For those who have learning disabilities also, the continuum of placement is important.

Level 1. Students are in regular classrooms functioning appropriately without any specific educational services. This level includes assessment services, monitoring, observation and follow-up.

Level 2. Students with handicaps function appropriately in the regular educational program with the assistance of special education supportive services being provided to the classroom teacher.

Level 3. Students with handicaps functioning appropriately in a primary placement in a regular education program, but needing direct service assistance from special education personnel.

Level 4. Students with handicaps functioning appropriately with a primary placement in a special education program.

Level 5. Students with handicaps functioning appropriately in primary placement in a special education program at a nonresidential school for children and youth who are handicapped.

Level 6. Students with handicaps functioning appropriately in a primary placement in a special education program in a residential facility for children and youth who are handicapped.[143]

The idea of placing disabled students, retarded or non-retarded, in a class with normal children for most of the day is a new and overpowering one. It is felt by some that mainstreaming is one of the best ways to integrate children. However, in some cases it may not be the best for all children.

When disabled children go to school, they must work with people they have never seen before and encounter experiences which may seem threatening. Socialization may become a difficult problem to deal with. In many cases, these children will not be accepted, creating a problem which children, teachers and parents must deal with realistically. It is important for teachers to realize that there will be more children with neurological problems in schools in the future because children are being properly diagnosed and helped by the more insistent parent-support groups.

More insight into the experiences of the child might provide the teacher with a better basis for assessing abilities. This would also make it easier for the teacher to interpret observations of the child, rather than basing assessment on test scores alone. Many things interact to build and develop the intellectual abilities of the child. "The broader the experience, the greater the individual's intellectual and behavioral range," commented Dr. William Cruickshank, a noted educator and writer.

Learning centers and resource rooms provide the place for children to get the extra time and attention which they need to work within the public schools. The teachers in these centers have had specialized training which better enables them to work with students with deficiencies. As mentioned earlier, some children need even more assistance than these centers can give, and they may need to be in special schools.

As noted in the Vocational Rehabilitation Act of 1973, the assumptions mainstreaming rests upon are as follows:

(1) "It is assumed that the special classroom is an isolating experience for retarded children. When in fact, the regular classroom may be even more isolating if not handled correctly.
(2) "These children are better able to achieve, both academically and socially at a level commensurate with their abilities when they are exposed to models whose achievement in both areas is more expert than their own.
(3) "The regular classroom bears a great resemblance to the 'real world' with which these children cope than does the protected classroom.
(4) "Exposure to disabled children helps other children to understand and accept them."[144]

Whether these assumptions are true or false must be proved in the schools. It's going to be very interesting to watch and see how effectively mainstreaming works.

A Philadelphia physician offered these words of encouragement and warning: "I feel that the problem will be corrected to some extent by mainstreaming the disabled child; however, I am fully aware that this will produce innumerable problems, not only for the general public, but for the disabled child and the family. On the other hand, I can see the objection that parents have in regard to sending their children to public schools and appreciate their desire to have their children treated in the environment that offers their children special education. Yet, I feel that all this will come to naught unless the population as a whole breaks down their prejudice against the disabled child."[145]

*　　　　　*　　　　　*

V

Employment

A. HARD TIMES

"Epilepsy may be set off by seemingly insignificant actions. In my case, swinging a child by the heels while playing airplane set off an unforseen storm of seizures. My father lost his grip and I fell, hitting my head on the couch," Jack sighed as he slumped in his chair. "Recently, my mother also told me that I was born with a brain tumor."

At the age of thirteen months, seizures began to be a regular occurrence for Jack and have persisted unabated since then. He is one of a minority of epileptics who has remained uncontrolled for the major part of his life. He suffers from a combination of grand mal and petit mal seizures. When he was a child, his seizures sometimes numbered 20 to 30 a day. Recently, he was hospitalized for a short period of time when they returned to such a high frequency.

Jack has had other complications in addition to his seizures. When he was a small child, his parents were divorced and he was sent to live with his great-grandmother and his grandparents. Although they loved him very much and treated him like a son, he was never allowed to do many of the things other boys his age did. He could not understand the restrictions placed upon him. In school he felt his fellow classmates did not accept him. They often taunted him by asking him for a performance. "Show us one of your fake seizures, Jack," they would say. This only whetted his appetite for a fight, which in turn exacerbated his seizures.

In spite of these obstacles, his grandfather was able to teach him one important thing. He must stand up for his own rights in this world.

Although Jack's seizures have not been controlled, he has found some relief with the new drug sodium valproate. He is also on carbamazepine (Tegretol), phenytoin (Dilantin) and Messantoin. The large dosage of drugs cause him to be groggy in the morning; and he finds it difficult to be alert.

The problems which accompany his conditions seem to have greatly influenced Jack's outlook on life. His seizures have been such a problem that he has failed to hold any kind of job for any length of time. He has never gotten the kind of job he wanted and has never been satisfied with the work that he did have. This in turn, has made it difficult for Jack to get along with prospective employers. It has also resulted in a great deal of time spent in unemployment lines. At this time, unfortunately, he gives one the impression that he feels that he is "owed" a job.

"I do not want to continue to be put down because of my tendency toward seizures. Epilepsy is a terrible thing to have to live with when it is not controlled, or when you never can be certain when the next seizure will strike. In my case, my barber is afraid to shave me for fear that I might have a seizure and he would hurt me. However, the thing that is even worse is the attitude of some prospective employers. The belief that the epileptic is not able to do a good job prevents many people from hiring them. Actually they are better workers in many instances," Jack says.

Jack is dedicated to helping other people better understand the disorder. He has a strong conviction that too many employers still adhere to the myths which have existed for years that epileptics are bad risks and poor employees; they will cause insurance rates to skyrocket and will disrupt other employees. He wants to see these ideas changed.

*   *   *

Many employers do not feel that they can hire persons with epilepsy despite the evidence that shows how well they work. Some employers fear that persons suffering occasional seizures are accident prone and will raise their rate of liability insurance or will make them ineligible for workers' compensation. This is not true. Persons with epilepsy are generally dependable workers. In extensive studies[146] carried on in industrial workshops by Epi-Hab Center of Los Angeles, it was found that total time of 425 hours was lost out of 475,000 hours worked by people with epilepsy, or approximately one hour out of every 1000 hours.[147]

One of the objectives outlined by the Plan for Nationwide

Action on Epilepsy was to achieve an increase in the number of severely disabled persons with epilepsy in noncompetitive employment, from the currently estimated 4,000 in sheltered workshops in 16,000 either in sheltered workshops or in equivalent noncompetitive employment in industry by 1982.[148]

The vast number of epileptics don't want to work in noncompetitive employment. They want jobs of equal stature as any other person. More companies are hiring people and understanding their problems than has been true in the past. A definite feeling of discrimination, however, is still felt.

*　　　　*　　　　*

B. DISCRIMINATION IN EMPLOYMENT

Fifty to eighty percent of decisions to hire are based on interviews. And interviewers unfortunately see prospective employees through their own prejudices which vary according to their outlook. The feelings a person has regarding specific disabilities can be a factor in their desire to hire people. Likewise, other individual characteristics can threaten the persons getting the desired job. The following stories of discriminatory hiring were related to me by R.J.

"Once, while talking with a woman who was interviewing prospective typists, I was shocked at the things which turned the interviewer off.

"Two ladies came in to take the interview. Both were intelligent and excellent typists, quite fast and accurate. The first lady had ravishing red hair and purple fingernail polish. When she had left, the interviewer turned to me and commented. 'Did you see those fingernails? I could not have anyone in *my* office with purple fingernail polish!'

"The second lady had just begun to type when she suddenly jumped up and asked to be excused. She had left her keys in the car, unlocked. The interviewer sneered, 'What a brain!' My friend wanted to ask her if she had ever left her own car unlocked with the keys in it.

"Both applicants were eliminated from competition because the interviewer did not like something about them. They were out of a job, even though they could do the work."

Just as these prejudices on the part of the employer prevented the hiring of these individuals, so prejudice against epileptics has prevented their hiring. For this reason, people are often reluctant to state that they have seizures, especially if it is under control and not obvious. Unfortunately, many employees have lost their jobs within two or three months if their employer was not informed of the possibility of seizures.[149] Of a group of successfully employed persons with epilepsy, fifty percent had not revealed their disorder at the time of employment and twenty-five percent had continued to keep it hidden from their employers.[150] The average employer will not hire a person he knows has had a seizure within one year.[151]

The social stigma which accompanies epilepsy can be more of a problem at times than the seizure condition itself. Unenlightened employers may fear that other employees will not wish to work with someone who has epilepsy. In some cases, a negative attitude on the part of the employer may even be a result of "oversell" by the vocational counselor. Persons with epilepsy suffer from stereotyping in the workplace and elsewhere.

Gallop polls taken at five year intervals from 1949 through 1979 show a growing acceptance of persons with epilepsy. This was demonstrated in the increased awareness of epilepsy shown in questions regarding: 1) parents allowing their children to play with epileptic children; b) declining percent of people feeling that epilepsy was a form of insanity; c) increasing percent of people feeling that epileptics should be employed.

Even with this increase, 6 percent of people asked still objected to their children playing with epileptics. Eighteen percent would forbid their children from marrying persons with epilepsy. Three percent still believe epilepsy is a form of insanity. These figures were based on interviews with adults, 18 or older, in more than 300 areas in the United States.

Although the nation as a whole has become more accepting of people with this disorder, the South, followed closely by the West, has shown the largest increase in favorable attitudes toward employment over the past thirty years. The South increased by 46 percent from 1949; followed by the West at 34 percent; the Midwest at 26 percent and the East at 25 percent.[152]

As people in both lay and professional societies work together toward educating the public, a more understanding people is evolving. Improved seizure control, employment by major industries of individuals with histories of seizures, and more reasonable legal regulations concerning immigration, marriage and operation of motor vehicles have helped to give a better, more positive impression of people with epilepsy.[153]

Sec. 503/504 of the Vocational Rehabilitation Act of 1973 was designed to provide needed employment on notice to disabled individuals and to forbid job discrimination solely on the basis of medical hardships unless some safety hazard is involved [Subpart B-504-84-41]

1. No qualified handicapped person shall on the basis of the handicap, be subjected to discrimination in employment under the program or activity to which this part implies.
2. A recipient that receives assistance under the Education for the Handicapped Act shall take positive steps to employ and advance in employment qualified handicapped persons in programs associated under the Act.
3. A recipient shall make all decisions concerning employment under any program which insures that discrimination on the basis of the handicap does not occur or may not limit, segregate or classify applicants or employees in any way that adversely affects their opportunity or status because of the handicap.[155]

The Rehabilitation Act of 1973 contained anti-discrimination and affirmative action provisions which inspired great hope among the disabled and their advocates. But since the law was passed, many unfavorable rulings have been produced. Today, there are enormous gaps in legislation which continues to allow for employment discrimination.[155]

Laws also differ between states. At the end of May, 1982, 46 states will have some sort of legislation or regulation concerning employment discrimination against the disabled. The only states that still have no such laws are Arizona, North Dakota, South Carolina, Wyoming, Delaware and the province of Puerto Rico.

The 14th Amendment guarantees that no state shall deny any person equal protection under the law. The 14th Amendment also provides that no state shall "deprive any person of life, liberty, or property without due process." These guarantees, however, apply only to public employment or to actions by the state or state agencies; they do not apply to private employers.

There are continuing efforts to educate employers. Agencies such as the Department of Economic Security of Vocational Rehabilitation (DVR) have helped in locating jobs for the disabled. While the DVR has received little public notice, its accomplishments should not go unnoted. Referrals are received from medical and social agencies, and the disability is then verified. A counselor from the DVR would then work with the client and a prospective employer to place the person in a job which relates to their specific needs and abilities. The counselor must be aware of the severity of the disorder as well as possible areas of placement. In considering eligibility of the clients for placement, the counselor secures information about the type of seizures, severity, frequency, warning period, length of seizures, personality conflicts, time of occurrence, medication used and apparent effect of the medication.[156] These factors are all important in determining the line of work most desirable for those with minimal or severe disorders.

Effective placement requires highly individualized assessment. If epilepsy makes it difficult for the client to keep a job, the DVR attempts to adequately prepare the client for his position and to make the employer aware of his specific needs.

If the job is done properly, an employer's reservations about hiring a person with epilepsy can be overcome. A large part of DVR's job is to determine the best possible field for the individual. If problems have not been dealt with before a person with epilepsy is hired, then the problems often multiply. It is important for counselors to periodically reassess the client's situation in order to solve problems which might evolve.

People with psycho-social problems should contact the Department of Economic Security of Vocational Rehabilitation. A physical exam will determine if they are eligible. Often a counselor can detect possible areas of difficulty in the initial interview. These problems must be dealt with in order to get suitable employment. DVR may recommend psychiatric treatment, and if there are psychiatric problems that are a barrier to employment, they assist the client in getting psychiatric treatment. Following this treatment, they generally begin vocational rehabilitation planning which can often be very effective. Together the individual and the counselor select the proper job goal. They may need job tryouts and evaluations to make a good selection. If further training is needed, it will be provided. If all that is needed is placement, this will be provided to the person once he is on the job. When work is successful, the DVR steps out of the case. DVR is active in all states.

Companies receive tax credits of $3,000.00 under the Target Job Program when they hire someone who is disabled.[157]

The Epilepsy Foundation of America's Training and Placement Service (TAPS) is another agency which deals specifically with job placement of disabled persons with epilepsy. TAPS is a national program aimed at increasing the employment opportunities of people with epilepsy.

In 1976, The Epilepsy Foundation of America, concerned with employment and underemployment of people with epilepsy, submitted a proposal to the Department of Labor (DOL) to establish a national program to increase employment opportunities for persons with epilepsy. The DOL funded the program and created TAPS. It is funded on an annual basis and continues in the five original cities: Portland, Atlanta, Minneapolis-Saint Paul, San Antonio and Cleveland. Another center was opened in Boston in 1977. Additional satellite programs exist in Portland, Maine, Los Angeles, Puerto Rico, Washington, D.C. and Miami.

The objective of TAPS is to provide on-the-job training (OJT), placement services and job development for persons with epilepsy between ages 14 and 65. From the program's inception, the involvement and participation of the private sector has been vital. Employers who have worked with the program range from Fortune 500 companies such as Control Data and AT&T, to small local businesses. Services provided for program participants include job seeking and job retention skills training, individual and group counseling, job finding clubs, referral, placement and follow-up. The TAPS approach to the employment problem has allowed the program to surpass its placement goals each year. As of May 1981, TAPS had assisted over 6,641 individuals with epilepsy and placed 3,419 of them in suitable employment.

A high percentage of people with epilepsy are capable, competent and eager workers. When problems arise that adversely affect the individual's outlook, TAPS attempts to provide skills which build self-esteem and self-confidence.

One half of the first 160 hours and one-fourth of the second 160 hours that the person spends receiving on-the-job-training is paid to the hiring company by TAPS. It has been estimated that for every $1 spent in the TAPS program, a return of $2 is achieved through productive individuals earning money which is eventually taxed by the government.[158]

Medical records are made available to employers by TAPS. While it generally isn't necessary for fellow employees, employers have the right to know about epileptics. Otherwise, they may hire people for tasks which could prove dangerous to the individual and/or the company. This is nothing more than a minimum safety measure. The following cases should give further insight. Some are factual, some are not.

1. Oscar, in his endeavor to get a job to repay the down payment on his house, signed up with a construction firm. He did not list epilepsy as a disorder because he was afraid that he would not get the job if he did so. While working on the construction job, five flights up, he had a grand mal seizure and fell to the ground. Landing on cement, he sustained a concussion which resulted in high hospital bills. Although the company paid the majority of the bills, he was forced to leave his job. Had he told the truth, he might have been placed in a different area with the same company, perhaps in the section dealing with planning or with mixing the cement, for example. He would still be in good physical condition and he would have less trouble getting another job, (if and when he applies for another job.) The fact that he has been fired from one job in which he did not list his

disorder as a factor will certainly be an impediment in his success in landing a second job. This should be underscored.

2. In contrast, Rex applied to a data processing firm for a job in the computer field. He talked with the person in charge of hiring disabled persons and explained that although his epilepsy was not completely controlled, he had not had a seizure in 8 months. He was hired on a trial basis. He did his best to do a good job and make his superiors feel that he was capable of doing the work. After four months he had a mild seizure, but because his employers and fellow workers had been alerted to this possibility, they were much more supportive and understanding and no problems arose. He continued to work for the company and improve his position.

These are examples of people who had epilepsy when they sought employment. What about the person who is already employed and suddenly develops epilepsy? He may suddenly find himself in a job which he is not able to continue. All people who work and have epilepsy face the problem of promotion. The stigma which has been attached to the disorder causes some employers to intentionally fail to promote deserving employees. In other cases, the new jobs may be jobs which would be affected by their problem.

Rick Duran won his battle against job discrimination in the Tampa Police Department. After having satisfactorily completed his tests and applications, he was told in 1975 that he could not take the medical examination because he had, at one time, had epilepsy. Under local law his history of epilepsy disqualified him from the job.

Rick, now in his early thirties, had not had a seizure since he was twelve years old. He filed a suit against Tampa and the Civil Service Board under Section 504 of the Vocational Rehabilitation Act of 1973. The court held that the city discriminated unfairly against him because of his apparent disability. [*Duran vs. City of Tampa*, 430 Fed. Supp. 75 (M.D. Fla 1977)].[159]

Duran's attorney said that the ruling was "extremely significant because it shows that just because someone has a history of a handicap, they cannot be denied public employment."

In Wisconsin, a state appellate court ruled that under its state law, once an employee has established that the sole reason they were not rehired was because they developed seizures, the burden of proof that the firing was not discriminatory is upon the employer. [*Chicago & Northwestern Railroad v. DILHR Labor & Industry Rev. Comm.*] Wisconsin law contains an exception where the employee is unable to perform at the standards set by an employer due to disability.[160]

In Iowa, a cafeteria worker, who was fired after having one seizure while working at the cash register of a lunch counter, is in the midst of an appeal of her claim. She won her case before the state Civil Rights Commission. The state trial court overturned the Civil Right Commission decision and found that epilepsy was related to her ability to perform the job and that not having epilepsy was a *bona fide* occupational qualification. This case is now in appellate court.[161]

There is a growing awareness on the part of employers that people with disabilities such as epilepsy are not the problem they were once thought to be. Companies are hiring people for their abilities, rather than rejecting them on the basis of their disabilities. Employers must learn to hire people regardless of their own personal bias. More legislation is being enacted to ensure the employees' rights and to establish fair hiring policies.

In 1971, Judge Warren Berger drew this analogy from Aesop's fables:

> "Congress has now provided that the tests of criteria for employment may not provide equality of opportunity merely in the sense of the fabled offer of milk to the stork [in a shallow saucer] or to the fox [in a long-necked pitcher]. On the contrary, Congress has now required that the posture and condition of the job-seeker be taken into account. It has, to resort again to the fable,—provided that the vessel in which the milk is preferred be one all seekers can use."[162]

VI

Advocacy

A. TWO STEPS FORWARD AND ONE STEP BACK

Gregory Durham could not see the justice in finding himself "relieved" of his job because he had had a seizure. Of course, the employer had assured him that it was all in the best interest, a likely story.

In a recent decision, *Lewis vs. Remmele Engineering, Inc.* which was handed down in December of 1981, the Minnesota Supreme Court ruled that a manufacturer could refuse to hire an employee who had previously suffered seizures, even if their seizure disorder was substantially controlled. The court's ruling dealt a substantial blow to Gregory's efforts to gain employment.

The *Remmele* case arose because Gregory Durham had filed a complaint of employment discrimination with the

Saint Paul Department of Human Rights. In his complaint he alleged that Remmele Engineering had unlawfully discriminated by failing to hire him as a trainee in its machinist apprenticeship program because he had suffered seizures in the past.

In the late 1960's, Durham suffered his first seizure while in the armed forces. After a second seizure quickly followed the first, he was placed on medication. While medication seemed to control the problem, he was honorably discharged in 1968. Gregory suffers grand mal, with no aura or warning and a complete loss of consciousness. Since 1963, he has had only two seizures, both of which occurred when he failed to take his medication. The last seizure occurred in 1974. They have not interfered with his work or caused him to miss time at work.

Remmele manufacturers, Durham's employer, deals with special machine fabrication and precision diemaking. Machinists primarily operate large machines doing high-speed grinding, boring, and cutting of metal machinery components. Because of the work involved, safety guards cannot be placed on most machines.

The company's physician claimed that Durham could not safely perform machinist's work. A consulting physician concluded that Durham could not safely operate hazardous machinery or work above ground level. Since Durham could not perform his duties on such a limited basis, Remmele fired him. (Remmele had been aware of the fact that he had epilepsy when he was hired. In fact they even had another person working there who also had epilepsy.)

At the trial, a neurologist experienced in treating epilepsy stated that Durham's seizure disorder did not present undue risk and asserted that he was capable of performing ordinary factory work. (The neurologist had not visited the Remmele manufacturing site.)

The employer introduced contrary testimony from a physician certified and experienced in occupational medicine who had visited the company. This witness asserted that employment posed a threat to the claimant's health and safety. He based this position on the fact that Durham had suffered grand mal seizures which were not preceded by an aura. As to the possibility of future seizures, the witness stated that "even a lengthy absence of seizures does not increase the probability that one won't have a seizure again." The district court accepted this testimony and found that complainant's disability would pose a serious threat to his health.

In reviewing the district court's decision, the Supreme Court observed that an employer could refuse to hire someone whose disability "poses a serious threat to the health or safety of the disabled person." To establish that such a serious threat existed, the employer "must establish that it relied on competent medical advice, that there exists a reasonable probable risk of serious harm."

The court noted that the machinery to be operated by Durham was "extremely hazardous" and that he suffered from seizures which are unaccompanied by an aura and which can produce a total loss of consciousness. In light of the hazardous nature of work at Remmele, Durham's type of seizure disorder posed a serious threat to his health and safety, according to the Court.

The court did state that Remmele could not deny employment to all persons with seizure disorder; indeed, they noted that there was someone working at the company who had epilepsy. A number of variables, including the type and degree of seizure disorder and the nature of the work sought, must be taken into consideration before determining whether someone can be excluded from employment because of a disability.

Although this decision was limited to the types of seizure disorder suffered by Durham and the extremely hazardous work at Remmele, the ruling of the court is likely to harm the chances of securing employment for persons with epilepsy. Most importantly, the court did not find that the medication's control over Durham's seizure disorder significantly reduced the seriousness of the threat to him. As a result, job prospects may not be improved despite success of treatment.

The likelihood that other courts and employers may interpret the court's decision more broadly is another matter of concern. Persons with seizure disorders may be denied employment even though the work is not extremely hazardous as in Remmele.[163]

Cases such as this are prime examples of the need for legal assistance and/or advocacy such as that provided by the Office of Human Rights and the Legal Aid Society. Although other forms of advocacy are equally important, advocacy that deals with employment is perhaps the most fundamental. The legal advocates who worked with Gregory Durham on this case provided him with self-confidence and initiative. Although he lost the case, the importance of his ability to singly file suit is considerable. And without the assistance of OHR and LAS he would not have been able to do so. In order to change court decisions, we must first educate public officials and the employers as to the actual nature of epilepsy.

B. ADVOCACY AT WORK

The word advocacy means to support, to plead. It is a process that has been in continual flux for the past twenty-five years. Today, people have began to advocate for themselves. Twenty years ago the Federation of the Blind began to advocate for legal rights and full citizenship through self-advocacy. Persons with Mental Retardation continued to do this in the late '60s and '70s.

As deinstitutionalization became a fact and more people were released on their own recognizance, the need to educate the handicapped in self-sufficient living styles became an important political issue in the 1970s. Individuals accepted their role and worked towards the liberation of all of their rights. Young people wanted to be an active part of society. For the first time, they stopped taking ''no'' from anyone, and planned to work for the betterment of their lifestyles.[164]

In the past few years the number of advocates in one area has mushroomed. A great many parent groups now support parents of children with developmental disabilities. These groups have been especially helpful in improving school programs which give children the most assistance. Other advocates have helped make life better for parents and children by sharing their experiences; parents who have successfully steered their children through the problems arising from epilepsy are often able to offer comfort and support to other parents who must also face these problems. This type of advocacy also aims to achieve the maximum level of integration and acceptance of disabled children among society in general.

Advocacy is an ongoing process. The case cannot be closed and put away in a few hours. It is necessary for the advocate to put time and effort into researching the case, talking with the people involved, and providing realistic assurance. Aside from the parent advocate and the self advocate, other basic groups include the citizen advocate, the systems advocate, the self-help or consumer advocate and the legal advocate.

Citizen advocates assist in providing physical or emotional needs. They work on an individual basis with a few people and, in many instances, their services are provided on a volunteer basis.[165] Their actions may be as simple as going to a movie with a client or as complex as assisting people with educational and welfare difficulties. For example, they may go with the parent to a school staffing to discuss the child's placement in special programs or work with someone on welfare to make certain the person receives the proper amount of assistance. When the advocate accompanies the parent to a staffing, they do not tell the parent what to say. The advocate remains in the background as much as possible, providing direct assistance only when necessary.

One of the basic goals of the citizen advocate is to make life as normal as possible for the individual. As people become capable of taking care of their own lives, they need less assistance. This is not an overnight situation; a person who is coming out of an institution may need a little time to adapt to their new surroundings. During this interlude the advocate may assist them in fitting into the community.

Currently, more young people with epilepsy are going through school, finding jobs and making themselves part of the community than at any previous time. In the past, they were often institutionalized permanently because they were believed to be incapable of coexisting with normal people. In some instances epilepsy is accompanied by mental retardation; in these cases institutionalization may be necessary. But this is certainly not always the case.

Unfortunately, at the present time, disabled persons are viewed with fear, hostility or pity. They are often treated as "second class" citizens. Citizen advocates strive to help the public understand the disorder through speaking engagements, community awareness programs and other awareness programs.

Systems advocacy generally means working through a group or coalition to change laws or to develop new programs which meet the needs and desires of disabled individuals.[166] It has been modeled after small groups which has grown to form larger coalitions influencing national organizations. They are especially needed in non-metropolitan areas. Two important areas of systems advocacy are:

1. Making certain that social service departments are not discriminating against people because of their disability.
2. Defending programs that attempt to make life better for people. This is especially true of persons with multiple disabilities.[167]

As recently as 1981, in one of the Midwest's metropolitan cities, advocacy was used to provide a change in the zoning laws of the city so that a halfway house for young persons with epilepsy could be opened. Due to resistance by the neighborhood, it took almost a year in court to change the zoning laws so it could be put into operation. Advocate groups working in the community and with the legislation were instrumental in the opening of this home. Systems advocates focus on fundamental structural problems that enable them to work towards essential change.

Marie L. Moore, Director of United Cerebral Palsy Association (UCPA) National Advocacy Project launched in July 1972, has written that class or system advocacy in the area of rights for the disabled has included the following approaches:

- Initiating, influencing, and monitoring legislation affecting the developmentally disabled or those handicapped in other ways;
- Using a systems analysis approach identifying services needed and/or changes sought in the service delivery system from the clients' or consumers' perspective;
- Initiating, influencing and assisting in the development of new services along with the improvement of a diversity of services;
- Promoting the active involvement of a diversity of consumers (disabled adults and the parents of disabled children) in the planning, policymaking, and monitoring of services at state, county, and local levels;
- Providing technical assistance to establish consumer action groups in the use of appeal procedures; and development of action strategies, and similar activities;

- Using community organization processes to develop better communication and cooperation among agencies, organizations, and consumer groups.[168]

Consumer needs may also be assisted through systems advocacy. Services to assist in guaranteeing equal rights, employment, housing and legal decisions, as well as education and the creation of proper treatment centers, are only some of the ways in which consumers partake of systems advocacy.[169]

The role of the self-help or consumer advocate encompasses many things. It is based on the assumption that people with disabling conditions (the consumers) are best able to determine their own needs. Consumers are consulted, surveyed, studied and evaluated by consumer advocates and are involved in the planning of services.[170]

Legal advocacy is based on state law, state based regulations, Federal law and court decisions. Legal advocates assist people by providing advice on the rights of individuals with epilepsy. They are also involved in training people to better understand the disorder.[171]

There are fourteen major areas in which legislation outlines the human rights of persons with epilepsy. They are the following: driver's licenses, marriage, sterilization, workman's compensation, adoption, antidiscrimination, arrest/search, institutionalization, reportability, special education, state certification, state education, state employment and state identification.

Drivers' licenses should be handled on an individual basis. At the present time, only one year of seizure control is needed to procure a license, provided that the doctor feels it is wise. Laws have been enacted to allow the physician to contact the Department of Motor Vehicles and report if they feel that the person is unable to drive without being held in violation.

Arizona, Delaware, Iowa, Mississippi, New Hampshire, Oklahoma, South Carolina and Utah still have sterilization laws which apply to persons with epilepsy. It is the position of the Epilepsy Foundation of America that they should be repealed.

The employee injured on the job is entitled to workman's compensation for the disability resulting from their accident. To insure payment of these benefits, the employer is required by law to carry insurance or to prove their ability to be self-insured.

Second injury funds vary widely in coverage and application procedures, but courts have directed payment for persons with epilepsy in instances of on-the-job injury during a seizure. To qualify for second injury fund coverage, the employer is generally required to release information about the previous disabling condition of their employee.

It is felt, that when a person is hurt during an accident, and is unable to do the job for which they are trained, they should receive vocational rehabilitation services, including training and job placement, whatever is necessary to restore them to suitable employment.[172]

Arkansas, Florida, Iowa, Missouri and Utah still have laws that don't permit the person to adopt children.

Over one-half of the states now have antidiscrimination provisions for the disabled in one of the following areas: employment, housing, public accommodations, property ownership, and state supported education and services.

In eight states, The District of Columbia, Florida, Georgia, Minnesota, New Mexico, North Dakota, Pennsylvania, and South Dakota, legal or administrative provisions require law enforcement officials to search a person subject to arrest for emergency medical identification. These provisions help prevent persons from being arrested for presumed drunkenness or other erratic behaviour when, in fact, a medical condition such as epilepsy is the cause of the semiconscious or unconscious state.

Surveys show that 15 percent of the states inquire into a past or present history of epilepsy on applications for state employment. Data are not available on how many employers in the private sector make this request.

Over one-half of the states surveyed provide identification cards for citizens not eligible for a driver's license. These identification cards help in the conduct of financial and business affairs. It enables the person to have an identification card, like a license which allows them, in some areas, to use transportation facilities at a discount.

Advocacy for the developmentally disabled appears to be moving in a positive direction. In October of 1975, the Developmentally Disabled Assistance and Bill of Rights Act (PL 94-103) was signed into law, protecting the rights of persons with developmental disabilities. Since that time, people have begun to advocate for themselves. In order to insure the rights of people with disabilities and their need for better assistance, advocates work with the government officials, the school boards and the park commissioners. The epileptic should be aware that he/she has people who can work with them to solve problems which they frequently must face.

To be a strong advocate, it is important to realize that resources exist around the individual. If adequate support groups are not available, they may be built through organized effort. They can be created by learning more about the law, reading regulations and realizing those things that are important. Be inventive. Turn to such organizations as the League of Women Voters, Closer Look and the Epilepsy Foundation of America on the National level. Organizations within the community are the place to start. We must advocate for one another to be effective.

*   *   *

VII

A Personal View of Epilepsy

MY TROUBLE STARTED YEARS AGO

When I was two and a half or three years old, I fell off of my tricycle while riding it up a grass slope. It tipped over and I fell onto the cement sidewalk. I had played hard all day, but that night I began having seizures. My right arm would go up and my head would turn to the side as if transfixed. My eyes had a glassy look which frightened my mother who was watching me play. The following day she took me to a doctor, whose tests showed that I might have epilepsy. The cause was not pinpointed. Further tests indicated that I had probably been injured at birth as my delivery had been difficult and had required forceps. That, coupled with the recent fall, could have caused the epilepsy to manifest itself. That diagnosis was made over 43 years ago when less was known about the disorder, and even less accepted.

My grandparents urged my parents to bring me to Los Angeles for further tests. The idea of their granddaughter having epilepsy was appalling and they hoped that more would be learned through further testing. Dr. Fred Roberts was a heart specialist well known for his work in pioneering open-heart surgery. Some of his colleagues were leading men in the field of neurology. After carefully examining me, the physicians told my parents that I had epileptic tendencies which apparently had been aggravated by the fall. During my stay in California, I had no seizures whatsoever. I was sent home to Texas on Dilantin in 1942.

When I was about four years old, my parents took me to Texas Children's Hospital in Galveston, Texas where an EEG was performed in the hospital's hallway. The doctors packed me and the electroencephalograph machine in tow sacks. An abnormal EEG was recorded.

Epilepsy was not well understood forty-two years ago, even less accepted. The seizures I have had have been mixed . . . both petit mal and motorized. For some reason, my parents were told that I had only petit mal, the lightest type of seizure. These seizures are brief and often mistaken for daydreaming. They last for only a few seconds and usually cause no noticeable change in behavior. Such episodes may occur in any person, but tend to be more common in children from ages six to fourteen. After a seizure, the person resumes what he/she was doing, and may not be aware that a seizure has actually taken place. Petit mal seizures can change into different, more serious types of seizures in later years.

Anti-convulsants are usually effective in preventing these mild attacks, and in 1942 Dilantin was recommended. This drug caused my gums to become puffy and enlarged.

A DIFFERENT LIFE

By the time I was eight years old, my parents' life began to fall apart. When I was in the seventh grade, they were divorced. I wasn't doing very well myself. None of the medication that I was placed on seemed to work and the seizures continued. Consequently, everyone guardedly overprotected me; I was not permitted to do things which most children do unless I was under constant supervision. I loved to climb trees, but I was restricted from doing this, because my mother was afraid that I might have a seizure and fall. On the other hand, my father wanted me to have an opportunity to do the ordinary things children do when I was in grammar school. He seemed to understand better.

In 1950, I moved with my mother to San Antonio, Texas where I went to school at Saint Mary's Hall. My father remarried at this time and moved to Sugarland, Texas. I was torn between accepting and not accepting my stepmother. My mother was very angry with the world and turned to alcohol. This did not make life easier. I moved into the boarding school in the seventh grade. My father and his wife would visit on weekends. I wanted to like Jody, my stepmother, and eventually found her a good friend. My roommate, who was from Mexico City, had a falling sickness much worse than mine. I suppose the housemother assumed we would get along well. She was right. Peggy and I became good friends.

I returned to my grandparents' home in 1952 to attend high school. At this time, there was a great deal of inner turmoil within my grandparents' home. They did not really approve of my visiting my father. Grandmother would not allow me to walk to school or to participate in any sports which she felt would aggravate my "condition." I was taken to Houston regularly to see the neurologist who commented on one visit that my main problem was not the seizures, but my family's overprotectiveness.

I craved acceptance by my peers and my family. I had many acquaintances but few close friends. My father was happy in his new marriage, but my mother was in and out of hospitals for the next twenty years. She would return to visit at times, yet was unable to give the love and support which I wanted and needed. I felt unwanted and rejected. These situations aggravated my low self-esteem which in turn, added to my seizures.

When I went to college in 1956 I had to struggle to make my grades. I enjoyed learning, but I found it difficult to concentrate on the school work, partially because of the medications which I took. I tried to get by on less medicine in order to keep my head clear, but my plan backfired and I had more seizures. Only my determined struggle to succeed seemed to pull me through.

When I was a junior in college, I had a double major in education and Speech Therapy. The professor in charge of the Speech Therapy Department felt that I was not a good candidate for the field. Because my seizures were uncontrolled, she felt that I might frighten my students. She gave me extensive courses in Speech Therapy for a year. My grades were not exceptionally high. When I had a seizure while working with children, she advised me to leave school and take a business course. Begrudgingly, I took her advice. I went to the business school my father suggested to learn shorthand and typing. I felt that I had failed myself and my father.

At this point, I almost married. I realized in time that I would be marrying for the wrong reasons—just to get away on my own. I was living with my father and stepmother at this time in a small town just outside of Houston. It was Jody who helped me realize the real reason I wanted to marry.

Nothing was accessible unless you drove and at that time Texas law required that you must have no seizures for at least two years. I did not have a driver's license. Six months was the longest time that I had gone without having a seizure. So I had to try to learn to rely on other means of transportation. I found it very difficult to leave home. There were no close friends to ride with, only my family. To a person who is twenty-one, the feeling of being tied to another's wishes and actions is devastating.

That does not mean that I had never driven a car. I was a daredevil when I was twenty. Because I had to get to the city to go to school, I learned to drive and bought a car. Each day, I drove illegally into the city. Everything was just fine for a few months. Then, one day during rush hour, I had a seizure. I lost control of the car and careened across a six-lane highway. The car landed in a roadside ditch.

Miraculously, nothing was damaged. No one was hurt. My father, who was driving just ahead of me, doubled back and shut off my car's engine. The only thing I remember to this day about that incident is seeing white chickens sitting on a barbed-wire fence on the side of the road. Needless to say, there were no white chickens roosting on a Houston highway. It was an illusion or hallucination. I have never driven since.

In 1960, I returned to college and worked toward a degree in elementary education. I still had difficulty studying and passing exams. Medication continued to make me sleepy and blocked my memory. That winter, I slipped on ice and almost fell. [I had also fallen from a window-sill in my dormitory.] A companion thought something was wrong because of the way I walked. I did not realize then that I had fractured the femur bone of my left hip. I continued going to school, lost weight and could barely move around. Although the doctor insisted that I had no broken bones, during Easter vacation it was necessary to have extensive surgery on my hip. This was repeated three months later. I continued taking courses by correspondence and in 1962 received a degree in education. I was unable to do my practice teaching and obtain my teaching credentials, however. I have always felt that this was one chapter which was never actually closed; I have continued to take education courses.

In 1962, I returned to New England to live with my mother for a year while I taught in a nursery school. I was having difficulty with my hip and my seizures, so I went to Hawaii for a climate change and further schooling. I still wanted to earn my teaching credentials. I loved my mother, but I could not get along with her. At that point, I did not get along with either of my parents or my stepmother. Nothing that I did seemed to satisfy anyone.

After eight months of education courses at the University of Hawaii, I went to Honolulu Business School and earned a certificate in junior accounting. I later worked for the United States Marines accounting department. I enjoyed my work. The seizures were under control.

I still felt as though I should have continued with the Speech Therapy. I wanted to be in an occupation which would allow me to aid other people. The writings of William Cruickshank had particularly fascinated me. Job discrimination was worse for the person with epilepsy twenty years ago than it is now. I still feel it today, however.

MARRIAGE

I married Robert Schumacher, a Navy career man, in Hawaii in 1965 for the right reason. I was alone in 1968 in San Diego, California when our oldest daughter, Norma, was born. Bob was in Vietnam.

Just before Norma arrived, Michael, Bob's son, his younger brother and his mother visited me. I took them all over San Diego before I went to the hospital. At the time, Michael was ten and Neil was eleven. I had never had any children or my mother-in-law visit in my home and this was definitely a new experience. I went into the hospital eighteen days early and stayed until Norma made her appearance. Bob's mother took the boys back to South Dakota.

Norma's delivery had been difficult. Because of her breech position, it was necessary to break her clavicle to deliver her. The fact that I had seizures, as well as a bad hip caused the doctors to use light anesthesia. She seemed healthy, but for the next six weeks I bathed her with one arm firmly strapped to her body.

I began working on a course in fiction writing to give me something to do while the children were still little. I wanted to find an avocation which I enjoyed while enabling me to release the stress on my life. Stress triggers my seizures. The course had been beneficial. I have enjoyed it.

The summer of 1968 was a difficult time. Bob had just returned from Vietnam and had not really become acquainted with his daughter when we were transferred to New London, Connecticut. On our way to our new home, we stopped and visited with my family in Sugarland, Texas. The stress was too much. I had fourteen grand mal seizures in fairly rapid succession just after we arrived. My stepmother put me to bed and cared for Norma until I came to my senses. She told me later that I had walked around in a daze for three days following the attack. I had acted as if I did not know what was going on. I talked, but I made little sense. I remember none of it.

The doctors in New London decided that I had developed psychomotor epilepsy. In some people, petit mal changes and becomes a different, more severe form of epilepsy in later years. My epilepsy had changed; I began to have multi-types of seizure.

I developed an addition to my epilepsy. When I have

extremely bad seizures, I speak fluent Spanish. The only explanation for this that I can find is the length of time that I spent rooming with Peggy. This ability to speak Spanish came as a startling realization to my husband.

In 1970 we were blessed with two more little girls, twins, Malinda and JoAnna. When they were eight months old, Bob left again for Washington, D.C. on a mission to learn Vietnamese. The birth of the twins caused my hip injury to become unbearably painful, this in turn aggravated my seizures. Hip surgery was considered in June, 1971. The bone specialist decided at the last minute not to operate.

In December Bob returned for three months before leaving for Hawaii. His orders had been changed and he did not go to Vietnam. We joined him in November of 1972. During the time that we lived at Barber's Point Naval Air Station, I experienced many severe seizures. Everything was in walking distance, so I did a lot of walking. Frequently, I would lose consciousness and fall in some person's backyard. The children would scream and run for a neighbor, who would call the ambulance from the near-by dispensary to come after me. This happened so many times that whenever my friend Minne heard the ambulance pass her house, she would comment: "There goes Nancy again."

People were very kind and always took care of the children until I came out of the seizure and returned home. My first comment on waking up at the dispensary would always be: "Where are my children? Are they all right?" I was always assured that they were in good hands. That helped.

Bob was never very concerned about my seizures. He felt

that they were a part of my personality which had to be accepted and dealt with. He still makes light of them. However, he can detect the onset of a seizure sometimes before I can by the look in my eyes, or the attitude I have. In some cases, I have been known to be extremely edgy just prior to a seizure for two or three days. Like most women, this is always exaggerated around the menstrual period. Bob has never allowed me to use my seizures or my hip as a crutch. He contends that I am capable of doing anything that I want to do.

While living at Barber's Point, I was constantly trying new types of medication. Rarely did anything work. In 1975, I was placed on carbamazepine (Tegretol) and primedone (Mysoline). My reactions were fast, and I liked the alertness I felt. In fact, I was quite independent. I began to believe that someday I might actually be able to drive. We left Hawaii in July of 1976. After we had returned to California and were driving through the mountains on our way to South Dakota, I had a versive seizure without losing consciousness. This was the first time that I had had a really bad seizure in almost a year and I had never had one without losing consciousness. Bob kept hitting me, trying to bring me out of it. I wanted to tell him to quit . . . it wouldn't do any good. But no words came out, only the horrible guttural sounds of the seizure. Luckily, I was wearing my seat belt, so when my body turned in the seat and I tried to open the door, I was unable to get out.

When we got to South Dakota, we stayed for a month and visited. Then we went on to Minnesota. All that fall, I felt very tired. For a while, I blamed the change of climate and circumstances for my lack of energy. Bob had retired from the U.S. Navy and we were in a new home in a new state. My seizures, which had almost come to a standstill, resumed. The family doctor ordered blood tests constantly. When he discovered that I was dangerously anemic, he contacted my neurologist. Sitting in the office of the neurologist, I realized that the medication, which had seemed so helpful in the past, was the problem. Wanting to cry, but feeling it would be better to smile, I looked at the physician and asked, "What next?"

"No more Tegretol," was his reply. "Your white blood count is dangerously low. For you to continue on this drug would lead to a dangerous form of anemia which could be fatal. This drug can be dangerous and it can work wonders. For you, Mrs. Schumacher, it has been both."

"I can't go off of the drug 'cold turkey'." I protested.

"You have no choice," was his reply.

Ordinarily if a problem arises, a person is eased off of the medication, however, when on that January day in 1977 the doctor withdrew me completely from the drug, several grand mal seizures struck me the same day and I was exhausted by nightfall. At six o'clock in the evening the neurologist called to give instructions on what drugs I would be on. When I tried to talk, I could not carry on a coherent conversation. He was forced to explain to my husband which drug was prescribed for me. The headaches which followed the seizures left me feeling miserable for the next few days. I was emotionally drained. My left leg was very sore because of the cramps it always developed after hard seizures.

For the next two weeks, my body tingled constantly, and almost collapsed from time to time during the day. My hands grew numb, and it became difficult to do simple tasks, such as beating cake batter. That really scared me. I had never had any part of my body become numb. Several times while shopping, I had to hold onto the grocery cart for fear that my legs would collapse. They felt rubbery. The medication which the neurologist had prescribed caused these unexpected problems. In spite of my strange feelings, I felt in good spirits. The drug that I was on is noted for giving a sense of euphoria to some individuals. When the neurologist realized that it was not working properly, he discontinued it and left me on Mysoline alone.

My body acted as it if had a mind of its own. I was never certain what would happen next. Although I was extremely tired and shaky, everything that needed to be done was done. The wash . . . the supper . . . the dusting . . . the children off to school . . . were all taken care of in their respective order. Bob left early for work as always. I was solely responsible for doing the tasks which housewives are expected to do. Everything went off as it should. I still wonder how or why I was able to keep going.

The neurologist tried several combinations of drugs that spring without success. I continued to take Mysoline alone. I remained on this drug alone for one and one-half years. It helped somewhat, but I don't recall falling against a cement building during a seizure in downtown Minneapolis. Someone was kind enough to assist me into the nearby building. The medical alert emblem which I wore around my neck made them aware of the problem I was having. Since it was winter and in the middle of a snowstorm, I was doubly grateful for the assistance. Just after this, in 1979, sodium valproate was legalized. I was placed on this drug in conjunction with Mysoline. Even this combination was only moderately successful. By this time, I was having multi-type seizures and symptoms which included petit mal, versive, Jacksonian, grand mal, psychomotor and complex partial and many others.

During the summer of 1979 I was still recovering from the total hip surgery which I had had that spring. In July my hair began to come out in handfuls. Someone suggested that it might be a result of the anesthesia used in the operation in conjunction with the drug sodium valproate.

Adverse effects of sodium valproate include hair loss and weight gain. In August the drug was increased, yet the seizures remained controlled. By February of 1981, I had decided that the drug really didn't work properly. I was still losing hair and gaining weight. This was depressing. Even though I realized that it would be risky, I eased off of the sodium valproate and remained on the Mysoline. I was feeling really good. I felt as though I were losing weight, then bingo. On March 13th (which WAS A Friday!) I had six grand mal seizures. One occurred every hour beginning at midnight. The following day I had another. In one of these seizures, it seemed to me that the world was completely purple. I seemed to be progressing through a maze. This was similar to the problems I had had in 1968. This time, Bob force fed me my medication until the seizures were under control. He felt that he could bring me out of it. (This is not recommended. When a person goes into status epilepticus, or a state in which one seizure follows another without stopping, a physician should be called.) I vaguely remember seeing the medication he gave me. It looked like an ant. (Some medications do resemble orange bugs.) I knew Bob, and I trusted him. He told me to take the medication he gave me. I did. After three days, I was no longer in a semiconscious state. The children said that I acted like a small child. Everything had to be done for me. Monday I was still confused and remembered only a portion of the telephone conversations which I had had. When I took my final examination at the University on Tuesday, I had difficulty writing and remembering the professor's name. Even on Friday, my memory had not fully returned. It was not back to normal for a week. This is the longest post-ictal or after-seizure recovery phase that I have ever gone through.

The seizures had a really adverse effect on my body functions. I felt as though I would come out of my skin on Sunday. It seemed as if my blood and muscles were outside of my skin. I had a very poor appetite. In order to bring me out of the seizure, Bob had insisted that I eat, as well as take the medication which he prescribed. Unfortunately, it was an old prescription which read 10 sodium valproate and six Mysoline. On Monday I told him that I felt that it was not correct. I could not remember how much I should take. When we finally contacted the neurologist, he gave us the correct dosage.

On the 26th of March I was still having difficulty remembering certain things. I had no trouble riding the bus and reading was getting easier. At times, while shopping, I would want to buy something, but couldn't remember what it was called or how to say the word. This was very embarrassing and scary. Gradually my memory returned. I did not continue at the University because I was afraid that the pressure from classes had been one of the causes for this. Instead, I began to draw. It was relaxing and enjoyable. Since then I have continued to use my art as a type of avocation and therapy.

I had relatively few seizures until the summer of 1982. These seizures were lighter, yet some of them occurred in very inappropriate places. I have almost drowned while swimming with the children. Only my daughter's quick action got me to a place where I was safe.

I was able to lower my medication once more in October of 1982. This time, I did it carefully and with the physician's assistance. However, in April of 1983, when I was down to one sodium valproate and three Mysoline, the neurologist discontinued the drug entirely. I had three days of status following this and was placed on Tranxene to take the place of the sodium valproate. During the time I was in a status situation, Bob said he thought that my heart stopped once. This combination of drugs is working and I have had only one bad seizure since May of 1983. Other changes in my life have relieved the tension that I had placed myself under.

WHAT IS A SEIZURE LIKE?

A seizure feels like an exploding electrical circuit in the brain. It can vary from almost unseen difficulties such as slight twitching to grand mal seizures in which the person falls and writhes, turning his head to the side and foaming at the mouth. The after-effect of this type of seizure is a terrible headache and a feeling of disorientation.

A warning of "aura" often preceeds the major part of an attack. The feeling of the eyes turning to the side, an unusual smell or a special sound can be part of an aura. Most persons with epilepsy are alerted by these early feelings. In my case, however, if auras do occur, there is only a split second before the actual seizure begins. This momentary feeling does not provide adequate time to prepare for the onset. Some doctors believe that the seizure begins when the aura starts.

During some seizures my head is pulled to the right and my eyes become transfixed upon my extended right arm. As my eyes follow my rotating arm, my entire body begins to turn. I cannot stop the turning. If I try to resist, which I sometimes do, it becomes worse. Sometimes, I spin around several times and then fall like a top. After the fall, I am told my body writhes.

For a long time, I would fight the fact that I was about to have this type of seizure. "I am not going to have it. I am not going to have it," I would say to my subconscious. If my head had started to turn, I would try to put it back where it belonged . . . straight ahead. This effort appeared to make the seizure worse. When I had a seizure in which I fell, my left leg would always contract painfully. The muscles within it were always very sore following the seizure. A horrible headache followed. After the seizure ended, I was confused and tired. I generally didn't remember anything that occurred during the seizure. Only when I was on the drug

Tegretol, I stayed awake during the entire seizure, which was an experience I would rather forget.

When you're having a seizure while you're awake, you're aware of the animal sounds that you make. They are strong guttural noises. If your head turns to the side, as mine does, you can't move it, nor can you talk, walk or carry on a conversation. If you lose your urine during the seizure, as I do, the warm feeling of urine running down your leg is quite upsetting as it flows uncontrolled down your leg and into your shoe. It is much easier to be completely unconscious of all this. Such a seizure can be embarrassing when it happens among strangers.

The fall of 1980 found me going to school at the University of Minnesota. Periodically, I would be waiting at the bus stop and suddenly realize that I had to catch the "Number 47", yet not know why or where I was going. I always managed to get onto the bus. Then everything cleared.

On one occasion, I crossed the street without ever realizing that I had done so. Still another time, I mistook the cars which were flying down Old Shakopee Road for bugs on their way to their homes. I was extremely lucky not to be hit on that occasion.

However, in November 1980, my luck ran out. I was not having a seizure. I was just crossing the intersection when a lady turned into my left leg and sent me flying. My knee was fractured and I was on crutches for the next four months. I had to stop courses at the University but returned three and one-half weeks later to take my finals on crutches. Since I had already registered for the winter term, I continued going to school on crutches. As you might expect, while I was on crutches and still in pain, my seizures escalated. I was allowing my body to become drained of energy.

At Christmas, Bob decided that we should go to Saint Paul to look at the Christmas decorations. While we were crossing the bridge which spans the Mississippi, the lights from the oncoming cars caused me to see colored spots. I began to have a seizure and tried to jump from the car. It was all that Bob could do to keep me in. This was a new type of seizure—a photogenic seizure.

In January of 1981, I slipped when I had a seizure and fell on my crutch on the cement entrance of a school. When I fell, every tooth in my mouth felt as though it were shaken loose. I did not come out of this seizure until I had been taken home by a friend and was in my living room. This was the closest that I had come to hurting myself during a seizure. Bob or the children have always taken sharp objects, such as knives, out of my hands when a seizure began. Later my grip is like a vice, and it is virtually impossible to break during the clonic segment of the seizure.

Our children have grown up with my seizures and have adapted to them. When I have seizures at home with the children around, they take me and pull me to the bed if I am really out of it. They are very attentive and careful. Malinda seems to be most organized, although JoAnna is very helpful also.

Of course when you have a seizure and are alone, you really don't know what to do. You have to hope for the best and try to remember the safety rules before you black out. (See page 14 for the list of safety rules.)

Since I have had almost every type of seizure which exists, I have definitely learned to temper my commitments. Although I enjoy working in the community, I have to be careful not to overdo things. When I allow myself to become too involved, I grow tired and this triggers seizures. Adequate rest and regular meals are essential for my good control.

Each patient is different and reacts uniquely to a particular drug or combination of drugs. Only through trial and error can appropriate medication be found. Overmedication can be as great a problem as not finding the appropriate drug. Some of the situations that I run across aggravate my ability to remain calm and controlled. In time, I hope to be able to find a combination of medications which will enable me to live a more relaxed life; a life which is free from seizures, or the threat of them.

Even as important as the medication, however, is the understanding spouse who can care for his partner when the going gets rough. The person who has someone who can emotionally fortify him/her is extremely lucky. I consider myself exceptionally lucky because my husband *knows what to do* and *does what is needed*.

Epilepsy has been swept under the carpet far too long. Information and personal experiences need to be shared on how to accept the disorder and those persons troubled with it. Many new breakthroughs are coming in science and medicine. It is important that the outlook of people also widen. It is imperative that proper education reach the general public in such a way that they find themselves losing their fear of the unknown—the falling sickness.

Those of us who have epilepsy can hope for even better medication. We can live useful lives in spite of our limitations. An attitude of thankfulness and appreciation for our blessings can enable us to do so. Epilepsy is nothing which we should be ashamed to have. It has become my goal to live to the best of my ability. By finding my talents and using them, I am trying to overshadow problems which may arise. I make myself available whenever possible to educate others about the disorder. But most of all, I have learned to accept myself and my family's love.

*　　　　*　　　　*

Conclusion

Through telling my own story, I have endeavored to explain how life appears to an epileptic. The fact that we have to fâce many difficulties not unlike those faced by the general public lends credence to the fact that, essentially, we are no different from others. We laugh, we cry, we pay taxes and raise families.

I have talked at length about the three major types of seizures: grand mal, petit mal, and complex partial and their various parts. Their consequences and their treatments have been explored at length. As new drugs are discovered and new methods of treatment advanced, the person with epilepsy stands a greater chance of finding a means of controlling their seizures in the best and safest manner. First aid has been mentioned in an attempt to make people realize the ease with which a seizure may be handled.

Parents have added their stories in an endeavor to help other people better understand the problems which they have had to cope with in dealing with this misunderstood and feared disorder.

The legal rights of epileptics with regard to education and employment have been covered in depth to provide knowledge of what laws are available and what laws are still lacking. Employment discrimination and acquisitions of drivers licenses seem to create the greatest number of problems for the average epileptic. Through support and advocacy, people are gradually gaining a better understanding of themselves and are developing self-esteem which is so essential to a happy productive life. Today is not the time to blame ourselves if our children have the problem, or to blame ourselves if we have the problem. It is time to educate those around us and let others better understand what we are capable of doing in this world. Only through education and constant renewal of our abilities can we hope to put away forever the myths which have plagued individuals with epilepsy for so many years. The speakers' bureau of the various EFA agencies are an important part of this re-education program, for it is at the local level that we must begin to educate the populus.

References

Chapter I

1. Jones, W. H. S., *Hippocrates 1952–58*. Cambridge, M.A. Harvard University Press. The Leab Classical Library. n.d.
2. Gastaut, H., and Roger Broughton. *Epileptic Seizures: Clinical and Electrographic Features, Diagnosis and Treatment*. Springfield, IL. Charles C. Thomas. 1972. p. 3.
3. Solomon, Gail E., and Fred Plum. *Clinical Management of Seizures*. Philadelphia, PA: W. B. Saunders Co. 1976. p. 1.
4. *Ibid*. p. 4
5. Isaccson, R. L., *The Limbic System*. New York. Plenum Press. 1978. p. 210.

6. *Ibid*. p. 210.
7. Solomon and Plum. *op. cit*. p. 39.
8. Solomon and Plum. *op. cit*. p. 4.
9. Penfield, Wilder, "The Physiology of Epilepsy." *in* Pupura, D. P., J. K. Penry, and R. D. Walter, eds. *Advances in Neurology*. Vol. 8. New York, Raven Press. 1975. p. 19.
10. Iversen, Susan D., and Leslie L. Iversen, *Behavioral Pharmocology*. New York: Oxford University Press. 1975. p. 91.
11. Fincher, Jack, "New Machines May Soon Replace the Doctor's Black Bag." *Smithsonian* (Jan.) pp. 64–71. 1984.
12. *Ibid*. p. 68.
13. Table developed by Fernando Torres, Neurosurgeon, Comprehensive Epilepsy Program, University of Minnesota Hospital, Minneapolis, MN.
14. Actual experience which happened to me in March, 1981.
15. Solomon and Plum. *op. cit*. pp. 29–30. Biemond, A., *Brain Diseases*. Amsterdam: Elsever Pub. Co. 1975. p. 211.
16. Gastaut and Broughton. *op. cit*. p. 51.
17. Laidlow, John, and Alan Richens. *A Textbook of Epilepsy*. Edinburgh: Churchill Livingstone. 1976. pp. 19–26.
18. Netter, Frank H., *The CIBA Collection of Medical Illustrations*. Vol. 1. *Nervous System*. Rochester, NY: CIBA Pharmaceutical Corp. Case Hoyt Cirp. 1977. p. 80.
19. Laidlow and Richens. *op. cit*. p. 20.
20. Laidlow and Richens. *op. cit*. p. 210.

21. Gilroy, John, and John Stirling Meyer. *Medical Neurology*. New York: Macmillan Pub. Co. 1979. p. 350.
22. *Ibid*.
23. *Ibid*.
24. Laidlow and Richens. *Op. cit*. pp. 19–26.
25. Laidlow and Richens. *Op. cit*. pp. 19–26.
26. Jackson, J. H., *Selected Writings* Vol. 2. J. Taylor, ed. London: Hodder and Stoughton. 1932.
27. Williams, Dennis. "The Structures of Emotion Reflected in Epileptic Experiences." *Brain (29): 35–38. 1979*.
28. *Ibid*.
29. Gilroy & Meyer, *op. cit*. pp. 350–353.
30. *Ibid*.
31. Biemond, *op. cit*. p. 202.
32. Matthers. A. P. 1961.
33. Beaussary, M. and P. Louiseau. "Hereditary Factors in a Ramdon Population of 5200 Epileptics." *Epilepsia* 10:55–63. 1969.
34. Biedmond. *op. cit*. p. 233.
35. Isaccson. *op. cit*. p. 50.
36. Papez, J. W. "A Proposed Mechanism of Emotion." *AMA Arch. Neurol. Psychiatry* 39:725. 1947.
37. MacLean, Paul D. "Some Psychiatric Implications of Physiological Studies on Fronto-Temporal Portion of Limbic System (Visceral Brain)" *Electroencephalogr. Clin. Neurophysiol.* 4:407. 1952.
38. Williams, *op. cit*. p. 29.
39. Jackson. *op. cit*. p. 50.
40. Spratling, W. P. *Epilepsy and Its Treatment*. Philadelphia: W. B. Saunders. 1904. pp. 449–450.

41. Geaser, G. "Limbic Epilepsy in Childhood." *Journal Nerv. Ment. Dis.* 141(5):391–397. 1967.

42. Ounsted, C., J. Lindsay, and R. Norman. *Biological Factors in Temporal Lobe Epilepsy.* London: Spastics Society Med. Books Ltd. 1966.

43. Livingstone, Samuel. *Comprehensive Management of Epilepsy in Infancy, Childhood and Adolescence.* Springfield IL: Charles C. Thomas. 1972. p. 493. Minter, Richard. "Can Emotions Precipitate Seizures— A Review of the Question." *Journal of Family Practice* 8(1):55–59. 1979.

44. Veith, I. *Hysteria, the History of a Disease.* Chicago: University of Chicago Press. 1965.

Chapter II

45. Williams. *op. cit.* p. 29.

46. Laidlow. *op. cit.* pp. 19–26.

47. Williams. *op. cit.* p. 28.

48. Townsend, N. R. A. "Epilepsy A Clinical View: Dept. of Surgical Neurology (Western General Hospital Crewe Road, Edinburgh E #4 2X). *in* H. F. Bradford and C. D. Marsden, eds. *Biochemistry and Neurology.* New York: Academic Press. 1976. pp. 175–179.

49. Torres, Fernando. University of Minnesota School of Medicine. Neurology Department.

50. Anderson, V. Elving, Deight Institute, University of Minnesota.

51. Bannister, Roger. *Brain's Clinical Neurology.* London: Oxford University Press. 1978. p. 108.

52. Bleck, Eugene E., and Donal A Nagel. *Physically Handicapped Children, A Medical Atlas for Teachers.* New York: Grune & Stratton. 1975. p. 106.

53. Solomon and Plum. *op. cit.* p. 2.

54. Richards, C. D. "Observations on the Mode of Action of Anti-Epileptic Drugs." *in* H. F. Bradford and C. D. Marsden, eds. *Biochemistry and Neurology.* New York: Academic Press. 1976.

55. Biemond. *op. cit.* p. 233.

56. *Ibid.*

57. Long, James W. *The Essential Guide to Prescription Drugs.* New York: Harper & Row. 1977. p. 477.

58. Townsend. *op. cit.* pp. 175–179.

59. *Physician's Desk Reference.* 35 ed. Oradell, NY: Medical Economics Company. 1981. pp. 406, 684.

60. Townsend. *op. cit.* pp. 175–179.

61. *Physicians' Desk Reference.* 35 ed. *op. cit.* 527.

62. *Ibid.*

63. Long. *op. cit.* p. 515.

64. Gilroy and Meyer. *op. cit.* p. 39.

65. Ahmed, S., John Laidlaw, G. W. Hughton, and A. Richards. "Involuntary Movements Caused by Phenytoin Intoxication in Epileptic Patients." *Journal of Neurology, Neurosurgery and Psychiatry* 38:225–231. 1975.

66. Gilroy and Meyer. *op cit.* p. 39.

67. Townsend. *op. cit.* p. 279.

68. *Ibid.*

69. *Physicians' Desk Reference.* 35 ed. *op. cit.* p. 552.

70. Townsend. *op. cit.* p. 281.
71. Biemond. *op. cit.* p. 233.
72. Townsend. *op. cit.* p. 281.
73. Berg. Bruce, *in* E. E. Bleck and D. A. Nagel, eds. *Physically Handicapped Children, A Medical Atlas for Teachers.* New York: Grune & Stratton. 1975. p. 196.
74. Silverman, Milton *in Plan for Nationwide Action on Epilepsy.* Department of HEW. Public Health Service National Institute of Health. DHEW Publication No. CNIH 79–1115.
75. *Ibid.*
76. Dreifuss. Fritz L. "Use of Anti-Convulsant Drugs." *JAMA* 241(6):607–609. 1979.
77. *Physicians' Desk Reference.* 35 ed. *op. cit.* p. 914.
78. Gilroy and Meyer. *op. cit.* p. 363.
79. *Ibid.*
80. Silverman. *op. cit.* p. 402.
81. *Physicians' Desk Reference.* 35 ed. op. cit. p. 619.
82. *Ibid.*
83. Silverman, *op. cit.* p. 402.
84. *Ibid.*
85. *Physicians' Desk Reference.* 35 ed. *op. cit.* p. 619.
86. Long. *op. cit.* p. 534.
87. Townsend. *op. cit.* p. 281.
88. *Ibid.*
89. Commission on Classification and Terminology of the International League Against Epilepsy. Proposal for Revised Clinical and Electroencephalography Classification of Epileptic Seizures. *Epilepsia* 22:489–501. 1981.

90. Townsend, *op. cit.* p. 281.
91. *Physicians' Desk Reference.* 35 ed. *op. cit.* p. 1530.
92. Walker, J. D., R. W. Homan, M. R. Vasko, et al. "Diazepam in Status Epilepticus." *Ann. Neurol.* 6:207–213. 1979.
93. *Ibid.*
94. Leppik, Ilo E., Albert T. Derivan, Richard W. Homan, Jonathan Walker, R. Eugene Ramsay, and Barbara Patrick. "Double-Blind Study of Lorazepam and Diazepam in Status Epilepticus." *JAMA* 249:1452–1454. 1983.
95. Wilkinson, M. "Migraine-Treatment of Acute Attack." *British Medical Journal* 2:754–755. 1971.
96. Jeavons. P., and E. Clark. "Sodium Valproate in Treatment of Epilepsy." *British Medical Journal* 2:584–586. 1974.
97. Gilroy and Meyer. *op. cit.* p. 363.
98. Silverman. *op. cit.* p. 468.
99. Long. *op. cit.* pp. 400–401.
100. Gilory and Meyer. *op. cit.* p. 367.
101. Vajda, F. J. E., G. W. Mihaly, et al. "Rectal Administration of Sodium Valproate in Status Epilepticus." *Neurology* 28:897–889. 1978.
102. Lezak, M. D. *Neuropsychological Assessment.* New York: Oxford University Press. 1976. pp. 37, 60–61.
103. Torres, Fernando. University of Minnesota School of Medicine. Neurology Department.
104. McGovern, John P., and James A. Knight. *Allergy and Human Emotions.* Springfield, IL: Charles C. Thomas, 1967. p. 1.

105. Philpott, William H., and Dwight K. Kalita. *Brain Allergies: The Psycho-Nutrient Connection.* New Canaan, CO: Keats Publishing Inc. 1980.

106. Conversation with William H. Philpott, M.D., Oklahoma City, March 1981.

107. Philpott. *op. cit.* p. 301.

108. Speer, Frederic. *Allergy of the Nervous System.* Springfield, IL: Charles C. Thomas. 1970.

109. Interview with Ralph Somner, Ph.D., Director of Chileda Institute, La Crosse, Wisconsin, April 1981.

110. Sterman, M. B. "Biofeedback and Epilepsy." *Human Nature* Vol. 1, No. 1:50–59. 1978.

111. Somner. *op. cit.*

112. Finley, William W., Hoty A. Smith and Murray D. Etherton. "Reduction of Seizures and Normalization of the EEG in a Severe Epileptic Following Sensorimotor Biofeedback Training, Preliminary Study." *Biological Psychology* (May 2):189–293. 1976.

113. Lubar, Joel, and W. W. Bahler. "Behavioral Management of Epileptic Seizures Following EEG Biofeedback Training of the Sensorymotor Rhythm." *Biofeedback and Self-Regulation* Vol. 1(1):77–104. 1978.

114. Sterman. *op. cit.* pp. 50–58.

115. Quy, R. J., W. J. Hutt, and S. Forest. "Sensorimotor Rhythm Feedback Training and Epilepsy: Some Methological and Conceptual Issues." *Biological Psychology* 9:129–149. 1979.

116. Englehard, Loretta. "Awareness and Relaxation Through Biofeedback in the Public School." E.S.A. March 1978.

117. Comprehensive Epilepsy Program Educational Materials, A Special Epilepsy Treatment Unit, University of Minnesota.

118. *Ibid*.

119. *Ibid*.

120. Shooter, Eric M., and N. McKenna. "Genetics of Seizure Susceptability." *in* H. Jasper et al. eds., *Basic Mechanisms of Epilepsy.* Boston, MA: Little Brown & Co. 1969. p. 689.

121. Metrakos, Julius, and Katherine Metrakos. *in* H. Jasper et al., eds. *Basic Mechanisms of the Epilepsies.* Boston, MA: Little Brown and Co., 1969. pp. 702–704.

122. Anderson, V. Elving. Paper included in *Plan for Nationwide Action of Epilepsy.* Vol. II, Part II.

123. Hirsch, Jerry, ed. *Behavior-Genetic Analysis.* New York: McGraw-Hill. 1967. p. 137.

124. Shooter. *op. cit.* 689.

125. Kubler Ross, Elizabeth. *On Death and Dying.* New York: Macmillan Pub. Co. 1969.

126. Anderson, V. Elving, W. Allen Hauser, J. Kiffin Penny, Charles F. Sing, eds. *Genetic Basis of the Epilepsies.* New York: Raven Press. 1982.

127. Junz, D., and D. Scheffner. "Uber Epileptische Anfalle bei Kindern von Eitern mit Epilepsie." *Nervansarzt* 51:226–232. 1980.

128. Anderson et al. *op. cit.* p. 96.

129. Laundin, G., and A. Molier. "Views of the Question of the Sterilization of Epileptics." *Acta Psychiatrica Scandi.* Vol. 26:; 77–189. 1951.

130. Anderson. Paper. *op. cit.*

131. Interview with V. Elving Anderson, Ph.D.
132. Solomon and Plum. *op. cit.* p. 5–6.
133. Laidlow and Richens. *op. cit.* p. 69.
134. Interview with V. Elving Anderson, Ph.D.
135. *Ibid.*
136. Inhelder. B., and J. Piaget. *The Growth of Childhood Thinking from Childhood to Adolescence: An Essay on the Constructional Structures.* Trans. A. Parson and S. Miligram. New York: Basic Books. 1958.
137. Interview with V. Elving Anderson, Ph.D.

Chapter III

138. Aberson, Alan, Nancy Bolick, and Jayne Hass. *A Primer on Due Process: Educational Decisions for Handicapped Children.* Reston, VA: State-Federal Clearing House for Exceptional Children. 1920. Insert from a booklet from PACER which deals with Public Law 94–142.
139. "Epilepsy and the School Age Child." Comprehensive Epilepsy Program. University of Minnesota. 1977.
140. *A Primer on Due Process. op. cit.*
141. Stores, Gregory, Jennifer Hart, and Niva Pizan. *Inattentiveness in Schoolchildren with Epilepsy.* Human Development Research Unit, Park Hospital for Children 19:169–175.

142. "Special Education 94–142 and 503: Numbers that Add Up to Educational Rights for Handicapped Children: A Guide for Parents and Advocates." Washington, D.C.: Childrens Defense Fund. 1978.

143. PACER Booklet . . . levels used to distinguish children in Minnesota.

144. Reynolds, Maynard C., and Jack W. Birch. *Teaching Exceptional Children in All America's Schools: A First Course for Teachers and Principals.* Council for Exceptional Children. 1977.

145. Letter from a Philadelphia physician, 1978.

Chapter IV

146. Laidlow and Richens. *op. cit.* p. 364.

147. Anngers, William P. "Patterns of Abilities and Capabilities in the Epileptic." *Journal of Genetic Physiology* Vol. 103:59–66. 1963.

148. *Ibid.*

149. Barry, Stephen T. *The Mid-Career Epileptic: Problems of the Onset of Epilepsy in Adulthood.* Boston, MA: Epilepsy Society in Massachusetts. 1971.

150. *Plan for Nationwide Action on Epilepsy.* Department of HEW. Public Health Service National Institute of Health. DHEW Publication no. (NIH) 79–1115. p. 12.

151. *Ibid.*

152. Laveness, William, and George H. Gallup. Jr. "A Survey of Public Attitudes Toward Epilepsy in 1979,

with an Indication of Trends Over the Past 30 Years. Bethesda, MD: National Institute of Neurological and Communicative Disorder and Stroke, NIH.

153. Wright, George N., Fred A. Gibbs, and Shirley Linde. *Total Rehabilitation of Epileptics; Gateway to Employment*. Washington, D.C.: GPS. 1962.

154. Vocational Rehabilitation Act of 1973. Sec. 503–504 Subpart B-504-94-41. A Summary of Selected Legislation related to the Handicapped 1975–76. U.S. Depart. of Health, Education and Welfare. Federal Register Vol. 42. No. 46. May 4, 1977.

155. *Plan for Nationwide Action on Epilepsy. op. cit.*

156. Interview with counselor for Minnesota Division of Vocational Rehabilitation.

157. *Ibid.*

158. Taps Overview. May, 1982.

159. *Duran v. City of Tampa*. 430 Red. Supp. 75 (M.D. Fla. 1977).

160. *Employment Discrimination: Alternatives to Section 503 and 504.*

161. *Ibid.*

162. Seventh Circuit (Gregg v. DuPower) 403-U. S. Seventh Circuit 424. 1971.

Chapter V

163. Minnesota Developmental Disabilities Law Report. Vol. II, No. 1. March 1982. 1982. pp. 8–9. *Lewis v.*

Remmele Engineering, Inc. 314 North Western Reporter, 2nd series, pp. 1–4.

164. Interview with Mel Duncan, Advocacy for Change Together, Minneapolis, May, 1982.

165. Wolfensberger, S. *Citizen Advocacy for the Handicapped Inpaired and Disadvantaged: An Overview.* 1972.

166. Speech by Rebecca Knittle, attorney with the Legal Aid Society in Minneapolis, 1978.

167. *Ibid.*

168. *Plan for Nationwide Action on Epilepsy. op. cit.* Vol. II, Part 1, Sec. VII–XII, p. 638–642.

169. Knittle. *op. cit.*

170. *Plan for Nationwide Action on Epilepsy. op. cit.* p. 715.

171. *Ibid.*

172. *Ibid.*

Glossary

abortus   The product of an abortion, usually a fetus weighing less than a pound.

* **adrenocorticotiopic hormone**   an organic substance, secreted by the pituitary gland, which stimulates the outer portion of the adrenal gland; it is sometimes used in the treatment of infantile myoclonic seizures

* **akinetic seizure**   a type of seizure characterized by stiffening of the arms and a sudden falling forward. There are no jerking movements during its brief duration.

* **alpha rhythm**   a descriptive term used in EEG reports for waves which occur 8–11 times per second.

* **amino acids**   group of related chemical substances found in proteins.

† **amorphous**   a shapeless monster—having no specific orientation of atoms; in pharmacy, not crystalized.

anorexia nervosa   A psychiatrically abnormal condition in which the patient, usually a woman, eats so little that she becomes almost skeletal.

antiepileptic drug   A drug used in the treatment of epilepsy.

† **apperception**   Conscious perception and apperception; the power of receiving, appreciating, and interpreting sensory impressions.

† **ataxia**   Failure of muscular coordination; irregularity of muscular action.

† **atoxic**   not poisonous, but due to a poison.

aura   A premonitory feeling of an attack, usually of epilepsy

† **automitism**   The performance of non-reflex acts without conscious volition; called also automatic behavior.

* **beta rhythm**   A descriptive term used in EEG reports for waves which occur 11–25 times per second.

bradycardia   Slow rate of the heartbeat

brain waves   Changes in the electric potential of the brain as manifested by tracings made upon paper by electroencephalography.

† **Broca's ataxia**   hysterical ataxia

catalepsy   Immobility assumed by a person, characterized by rigidity of the body, lack of expressiveness of the face.

* **Cerebral dysfunction**   A term used to describe a child who is distractible, clumsy, and hyperactive and who has a short attention span. His ability to reproduce simple geometric figures or other tasks requiring perceptual motor ability is usually poor, but his memory for isolated events is likely to be amazingly good.

cerebral palsy   A motor handicap caused by an injury or malformation of the brain.

convulsion   A seizure, a fit, an involuntary contraction of voluntary muscles, i.e. those under control of the will, resulting in rapid, violent, spasmodic movement.

delusion   A false belief not culturally normal or common.

Dilantin   Trade name for diphenylhydantoin

diphenylhydantoin (DPH)   A drug used in ameliorating the symptoms of epilepsy.

* **dyslexia**   Inability to read at a level expected by age and ability in other areas of development.

† **double-blind study**   A study in which two variables are tested on two different sources.

dysrhythmia   Irregular electric brain waves on an encephalogram.

eclampsia   A toxic state characterized by convulsion in a pregnant woman due to high blood pressure or accumulation of fluid, often associated with coma (unconsciousness).

electrocardiogram (EKG or ECG)   A tracing on paper of the electrical potential of the heart.

electroencephalogram (EEG)   A tracing or record of the ''brain waves''—the electrical potential of the brain— used in diagnosis of several neurological conditions, especially epilepsy. The instrument is an enecephalograph. The study is encepholography.

episode   An event or happening.

† **EPSP**   excitatory postsynaptic potentials in each cell which will evoke all-or-none discharges. Neuronal hyperactivity which is fundamental to the process of epilepsy can clearly generate such synaptic insults.

febrile   Pertaining to fever.

fever convulsions   A convulsion associated with a fever.

fontanelle   In an infant, a spot on the skull not yet fused.

fugue   An unannounced departure and temporary disappearance of a person—when he returns he may say he has no memory of why or where he went.

gastric cirsis   A spell of intense pain in the abdomen sometimes with vomiting.

gastrointestinal   Referring to the stomach or intestines.

grand mal   Typical convulsion of epilepsy

† **hallucination**   Severe disturbances of perception in which nonexistent entities are seen or heard.

hydrocephalus   A condition in which there is an accumulation of fluid in the brain ventricles manifested in a substantially enlarged head with broadened forehead and often accompanied by mental retardation or episodes of convulsions.

hysteria   An emotional state characterized by uncontrolled emotion; also its conversion into a physical symptom.

hysterical   Pertaining to or due to hysteria.

* **idiopathic**   From an unknown cause

irascibility   quickness or fieriness of temper

* **IQ**   The score on a test of intellegence in which the child's performance is compared with other children of his own age. Ordinarily the value is expected to remain reasonably constant for a child (with-in errors of measurement) over a period of time. Formerly IQ was defined simply as MA/CA times 100 (Mental Age divided by chronological age times 100). In recent years it has been more prescisely defined for statistical purposes of the degree to which the received score deviates from the average of children his own age.

jactitation   Head tossing as in acute discomfort

‡ **kindling**   Refers to the effects produced by brief periods of electrical stimulation applied at regular intervals but separated by hours or days.

† **Lennox-Gastaut syndrome** (Myoclonic-astatic epilepsy) These children's immature brain shows a remarkable degree of excitability. There is a risk of status epilepticus developing from no detectible external or internal reason (p. 84 Jasper)

mainstreaming The practice of mixing together in an educational setting both handicapped and nonhandicapped children to the maximum extent appropriate. The act is predicated on this principle. The former will be placed in specific classes or separate schools only when the nature or severity of the handicap is such that education in regular classes even if they are provided supplementary aids and services cannot be achieved satisfactorily.

† **mediological context** An inhibition of the normal development of mental process.

mental retardation An inhibition of the normal development of mental process.

† **monotherapy** Therapy with one drug.

Moro reflex A neurological reflex produced in infants by striking the table on which the infant is placed, whereupon the arms fly upward as in an embrace.

narcolepsy A sudden and uncontrollable attack of sleep—its paroxysmal nature is apparent from its syndrome, sleep epilepsy.

neurosis A disturbance of mental or emotional function in one or more aspects of daily living without substantial loss of reality, unlike psychoses.

paroxysm A spell, or a sudden recurrence of a symptom; paroxysmal (adj.), characterized by paroxysms.

petit mal Momentary or other brief blackout—loss of

consciousness during which an individual stops what he is doing with no recollection of the blackout. Distinguished from grand mal, the classic convulsion of epilepsy.

phobia   An abnormal fear, usually of inanimate objects or surroundings that do not normally stimulate fear.

† **poly genic**   Pertaining to or affecting several different genes.

† **probands**   Propositus. The original person presenting with or likely to be subject to, a mental or physical disorder and whose case serves as the stimulus for hereditary or genetic study.

psychosis   A major mental or emotional disorder in which there is a departure from the normal aspects of acting, feeling and thinking, in which reality, perception, behavior, beliefs or attitudes are substantially distorted.

regurgitation   Bringing up food. Vomiting.

* **scan**   A test in which the accumulation by a particular organ of small amounts of radioactive particles is recorded. The kind of radioactive material is selected for the specific organ. Iodine, for example, is used for the thyroid.

* **scatter**   In testing, an inconsistency of a subject's scores on various parts of the test.

Sensory epilepsy   Epilepsy characterized by hallucinations of the senses—such as aberrant smells, sights, taste sensations.

† **sentiment du deja vu**   means that the environment suddenly assumes a very well known and familiar character.

† **sentiment de l'inconnu'**   environment becomes terrifyingly unreal.

serum half life   The time required for the serum to halve. (Textbook of Epilepsy p. 192)

single blind   A study using only one variable

* **status epilepticus**   Frequent and closely spaced recurrent grand mal seizures which do not respond to anticonvulsant medication.

* **steroid hormone**   A group of chemically related organic substances originating in certain glands in the body.

trance   A condition of somnolence or reduced consciousness.

§ **triple blind study**   When neither the patient nor the person administering the drug nor the evaluator of the study knows whether the administered drug is real or a placebo.

von Recklinghausen's disease   A genetic predisposition to a condition characterized by tumors of bones, muscles, and nervous system.

*Baird, Henry W. M.D. *The Child With Convulsions. A Guide to Parents, Teachers, Counselors and Medical Personnel*. Grune & Stratton, 1972

†*Donaldson's Illustrated Medical Dictionary, 25th Edition*. W.B. Saunders, 1974.

Alvarez, Walter C. *Nerves In Collision*. 1972, Phyramid House.

‡Pingham, Christopher, head of Statistics Department, University of Minnesota. Conversation held on June 26, 1986.

§Goddard, G.Z., McIntyre, D.C., and Leech, C.K. "A Permanent Change in Brain Function Resulting from Daily Electrical Stimulation." *Experimental/ Neurology* 25:295–30 (1969).

June 30, 1981

Ms. Nancy Schumacher
10236 Xerxes Avenue South
Bloomington, Minnesota 55431

Dear Ms. Schumacher:

My congratulations to you for being something of a
pioneer in the field of epilepsy and having the courage to
write a book which will help in the efforts of many who
are involved in bringing the facts about epilepsy to the
public. It is not an easy task to change the thinking and
misconceptions of this illness which have evolved over
the centuries. It is due to this length of time in which
epilepsy was not understood or properly treated that
legislation, both on the state and federal level, is needed
to familiarize the population with the truth about epilepsy.

In the past the legislature and governor have addressed the
needs of other disability groups in a variety of ways.
However, the rights of people with epilepsy have never
been addressed from a legal standpoint. During the 1981
legislative session I had the privilege of being chief
author of the bill which will establish an Advisory
Council on Epilepsy, a council which will report on the
status of programs, services and facilities for persons with
epilepsy in Minnesota.

At least one percent of the population has epilepsy. In
Minnesota approximately 80,000 citizens have epilepsy. Past

Minnesota law prohibiting marriage of persons with epilepsy was only one of about 60 laws which was discriminatory. Although the majority of these laws have been repealed or the language changed, the fact remains that the state government has done little to assure protection against discrimination. A state Advisory Council will identify these problems and needed services and will recommend needed research. The Council will communicate with agencies, the Governor and the legislature, ways in which these problems and discriminations can be alleviated.

Your book will serve as a source of information for people working with this illness, but more importantly it will give encouragement and inspiration to people with epilepsy in their efforts to acknowledge their personal situation. Truly, you are to be commended for your efforts to bring to the readers an enlightened awareness of the illness of epilepsy.

Sincerely,

(Signed)

Sam G. Solon, Chairman
SENATE HEALTH, WELFARE AND
CORRECTIONS COMMITTEE

SGS:bf

Index